# Secrets of Life Exte

Dedicated to the numerous researchers from all walks of science who have helped to bring gerontology to its present state of development, to the thousands of daring individuals who have been conducting experiments upon themselves with life-extension drugs, and to the countless laboratory animals which have involuntarily sacrificed their lives so that mankind could follow its pursuit of immortality.

# Secrets of

## A Practical Guide

# Life Extension

for the Use of Life-Extension Therapies

## John A. Mann

*Edited by Aidan Kelly, Ph.D.*
*and Dzintar E. Dravnieks, Ph.D.*

*Harbor Publishing, Inc.*
*And/Or Press, Inc.*
*1980*

The material herein is intended for information and study. The publishers and author advise any life-extension program be undertaken in conjunction with your personal physician.

Co-published by:   And/Or Press, Inc.          Harbor Publishing, Inc.
                   P.O. Box 2246                The Ferry Building
                   Berkeley, CA 94702           Room 321
                                                San Francisco, CA 94111
                                                Distributed by
                                                G.P. Putnam's Sons

Printed in the United States of America by the George Banta Co.

First printing: July 1980

ISBN: 0-915904-47-0

**Library of Congress Cataloging in Publication Data**

Mann, John A
   Secrets of life extension.

   Bibliography; p. 163
   Includes index.
   1. Longevity. 2. Aging. 3. Rejuvenation.
I. Title. [DNLM: 1. Aging — Popular works.
2. Aging — Drug effects — Popular works. 3. Longevity
— Drug effects — Popular works. WT120 M281s]
QP85.M34      612'.68      80-15479
ISBN 0-915904-47-0

Project Coordinator: Sebastian Orfali

Book and Cover Design: Bonnie Smetts
Cover Photograph: Charlie Jenkewitz

Manuscript Editor/Copy Editor: Aidan Kelly, Ph.D.
Developmental/Technical Editor: Dzintar E. Dravnieks, Ph.D.

Illustration Research & Development: Dzintar E. Dravnieks, Ph.D.
Illustrator: Phil Gardner
Molecule Illustration: Suellen Ehnebuske

Typesetting: Accent & Alphabet, Berkeley, CA

Proofreading: Bennett Cohen, Steve Murray, & Sayre Van Young
Index: Sayre Van Young

# Contents

# Foreword
## by Saul Kent

*Secrets of Life Extension* by John A. Mann is a valuable addition to the rapidly growing body of literature on the most important revolution of all time. As Mann points out, scientists have already begun to unravel Nature's secrets for health and longevity, and pioneering "longevists" are trying to take advantage of this knowledge. In doing so, they have embarked upon a fantastic journey that could, eventually, lead to the achievement of physical immortality.

Mann's major contribution to the revolution is the wealth of material he provides on the therapies these pioneers are taking in their efforts to extend their own lives. At a time when life extension is not yet considered a legitimate therapeutic goal by the medical establishment, Mann gives detailed, practical information on the vitamins, minerals, drugs, dietary regimens, and temperature-reduction techniques now under scrutiny as potential anti-aging therapies.

My only point of contention with the book is Mann's failure to include negative findings about certain compounds that tend to weaken the argument for their use as anti-aging therapies. For example, he fails to mention two animal studies which suggest that high doses of vitamin C may shorten rather than lengthen lifespan.

Unfortunately, it is difficult to evaluate current therapies because none of the studies conducted to date can be considered definitive. There have been no controlled, clinical trials to test the efficacy of potential anti-aging therapies, and relatively few lifespan studies in animals.

The primary stumbling block with regard to the testing of clinical therapies is the lack of a method to measure aging in humans. It's clearly impractical to conduct lifespan studies in humans because of the prohibitive length of the human lifespan.

Those of us who want authentic life-extension therapies for ourselves simply can't wait that long.

On the other hand, an effective battery of tests to measure aging would enable us to evaluate today's most promising therapies within a decade, and would aid immeasurably in the development of new therapies. Interestingly, the only way of validating such a test battery would be to use it to evaluate potential anti-aging therapies, with subsequent morbidity and mortality data serving as a guide to the assessment of both the tests and the therapies.

Several researchers are engaged in preliminary studies to develop test batteries to measure aging. Such efforts deserve large-scale financial support, as do all imaginative efforts to define the nature of the aging process. Out of such work will come the discoveries we need to develop and authenticate more effective life-extension therapies in the future.

Meanwhile, we'll have to depend on books like *Secrets of Life Extension* to satisfy our need for information on potential anti-aging therapies.

Saul Kent
Woodstock, N.Y.
author, *The Life-Extension Revolution*

# Preface

How would you like to live 120 years or more? It is now possible, and many people are already taking steps to attain that goal.

"Who wants to be that old?" you might ask. Not many of us care to hang around that long if it means being "old" in the sense that we have come to know the word. But what if you could slow down the aging process and perhaps even reverse it? What if you could look and feel like 30 when you're 50 or 60; like 40 when you're 70 or 80; and better than most people at 50 when you're 90 or 100? What if you could avoid the aches, ailments, depression, anxiety, energy loss, and mental and physical deterioration that happens to most people during what are supposed to be the "golden years" of life? In short, what if you could remain just about as vibrant and beautiful as you are today? Would you still turn down the chance?

This book explores what science has learned about the causes and control of aging, and examines the therapies that many people are currently using to preserve youth and extend the lifespan.

To understand what makes us age and how aging can be controlled, we will take a guided tour through parts of the body where aging is initiated. We will journey into several glands and organs that signal the body to age, and travel through the bloodstream to the immune system, the Jekyll and Hyde of the body that so easily switches from savior to saboteur. We will enter the microscopic realms within the living cells to take a germ's-eye view of their inner workings, and descend even further, into the world of atoms and molecules, where we can gain a simplified understanding of some of life's complex chemistry.

In our "fantastic journey," we will be introduced to some constituents of life whose names may be unfamiliar to anyone who is a bit rusty on high-school biology and chemistry. I will introduce them, and explain exactly what they are and what they do. They have precise names—such as catecholamine, hypo-thalamus, lymphocyte, mitochondria, embryonic fibroblast, decarboxylation, or dimethylaminoethanol—which we must use so that we know precisely who and what we are talking about. Do not let this precision make you think that this is a highly technical book, beyond the grasp of anyone with less than a Ph.D. That is certainly not so. Although we must use a few scientific terms to describe scientific facts, we do so for the sake of clarity, and present the information in language the average reader should have no problem understanding. If you happen to forget the meaning of a word, there is a handy glossary on page 169.

To help make our subject even more digestible, Chapter I, "The Life-Extension Story," gives a brief history of gerontology, the study of aging. In it we lightly touch on most of the material that is thoroughly explored in the subsequent chapters. If the reader has a scientific background, we hope that he or she will bear with—or scan through—passages intended for those who lack this advantage.

Gerontology is the scientific study of the causes and effects of aging, and of means of controlling or ameliorating these. Geron-tologists are the scientists who pursue this study. Longevists are not necessarily gerontologists, but are individuals who attempt to apply to themselves whatever is known about the control of aging. It is primarily the longevist to whom this book is directed.

Anyone who has been following the recent progress of ger-ontology is aware that the human race is at a unique moment in its history and evolution. Man, the longest-living mammal on Earth, is on the verge of extending his natural lifespan by at least 50 per cent, perhaps by much more. Scientists have already suc-ceeded in extending the lifespans of laboratory animals by means of several radically different drugs and techniques, a fact which indicates that there is more than one cause of aging. Some of these antiaging approaches are drastic, risky, or at least disadvan-tageous for human application. Yet others are essentially safe, and may be generally beneficial in that they promote life extension primarily by means of health extension. Even if they don't add years to one's life, they can add life to one's years.

Since most of these drugs can be obtained inexpensively and without prescription, thousands of people are now taking them daily. Some are using them intelligently, others ineffectively. Many may even be doing themselves more harm than good. Anything—even a vitamin—can be abused. Unfortunately, little or no information has been available on the human use of these substances. The scientific and medical establishment will probably continue to have no advice to offer on how to use these life-extension drugs until they have become standard prescription therapies; but that stage, for reasons explained in Chapter I, may not be reached for many years. Meanwhile, life-extension drugs are here, and people will use them. Before doing so, they would be wise to learn what they can about these agents, in order to derive the maximum benefits and avoid the risks of misuse.

Although some gerontologists are also longevists, in that they take life-prolonging drugs, most longevists are lay persons whose self-educations in this field have been obtained from conversations with other longevists or from the few books and magazine articles that have been published on the subject. Much of this literature gives excellent accounts of the history, present trends, and probable future of gerontology. Except for one of my own earlier publications, none of these writings touch on the fact that many people have already embarked on their own life-extension programs, nor do they detail safe and practical ways of using these drugs. * Because of this lack of information, many longevists have been using these drugs improperly, and are either deriving little good from them or are unwittingly causing themselves harm.

In this book, we will examine the pertinent facts about the known or suspected causes of aging, and about the drugs and therapies which longevists are now using in their efforts to control them. I hope that this book will help longevists to help themselves properly, so that their self-experimentation can go down in history as one of gerontology's noble and productive pioneering efforts, rather than as one of its occasional mistakes.

For more than five years, I have been experimenting with these substances, developing my own life-extension program, studying the work of researchers, and exchanging information and experiences with others who have been doing likewise. On the basis of existing scientific literature and our personal findings, we have attempted to discover optimal dosages and sensible ways to use these materials. I would now like to share with my readers what my fellow longevists and I have learned so far.

By offering this book, we are not urging the reader to use these therapies. We are simply trying to supply as much information about them as possible, so that those who already intend to use them may profit from both our successes and our mistakes.

Mark Twain once said, "Only kings, editors, and people with tapeworms have the right to use the editorial 'we.'" If I (or we) occasionally lapse into this practice, it results neither from tapeworms nor from delusions of grandeur, but simply from the fact that I cannot help feeling indebted to so many other persons for the information and ideas presented here.

---

* There are a few books which deal with some specific aspects of life-extension therapy. Among these are *Dr. Frank's No-Aging Diet*, by Benjamin S. Frank; *Slowing Down the Aging Process*, by Hans J. Kugler; and *Supernutrition*, by Richard A. Passwater. The latter two contain much good information on the use of megavitamins for maintaining youthful vigor. I discuss Dr. Frank's diet at length in Chapter 5.

# Acknowledgments

I totally lack experience in writing acknowledgments (I even sweat over simple thank-you notes). Although I have written almost two dozen books in the past, they were — with minor exceptions — one-man productions, at least in their initial editions. It has been a rewarding experience to team up with so many capable and creative people.

Some of the people who worked for or with And/Or contributed such a wide variety of essential creative functions that I do not know how to express my appreciation and recognition fully yet concisely. Aidan Kelly, for instance, did much more than merely a splendid job of editing; he also organized the strategy and structure of the book.

How do I even begin to thank Dzintar Dravnieks? He deserves some kind of medal. His devoted work as scientific and technical editor, coordinator, and research facilitator made me often feel that he was virtually a co-author of this book.

My feelings about Sebastian Orfali pass beyond gratitude. He did much more than simply act as publisher. He not only contributed much creative thought and effort to the shape and structure of the book, but also had to be the master-juggler walking the tightrope of a very difficult business, solving endless problems as they came up, and making decisions that ultimately turned disadvantage to advantage (I pause to multiply all this by the number of other books he has had to deal with similarly at the same time) — all this, while maintaining a sense of fairness, consideration, and concern for the needs of the author.

I also want to thank all the people at And/Or Press for their intelligent guidance, contagious enthusiasm, and persevering energy that brought my initial manuscript to its ultimate form as a book, particularly: Ryan Garcia, who did the initial editing; Phil Gardner, for creating graphics, illustrations, and charts; Bonnie Smetts, for creating the layout and design; as well as Leslie Strauss, Peter Beren, Linda Gibbs, Bill Alexander, and anyone else whom I may have inadvertently or through ignorance overlooked. I am also most grateful to Art Quaife and Gladys A. Sperling for the photographs they have contributed to the book.

A really complete list of acknowledgments could fill many pages, and would include the thousands of scientists who did the research work that I have merely written about. It would also include the names of nearly a hundred private individuals who have shared with me their experiences and personal findings during self-experimenting with life-extension drugs and related therapies. I do, however, want to thank specifically the scientists, physicians, science writers, and other very knowledgeable persons with whom I have conversed or corresponded, as well as those who offered a thought or two that led me to delve into issues that deserved further discussion. Among these are: Herb Gerjuoy, Ph.D., Senior Staff Scientist, the Futures Group, Glastonbury, Conn.; Paul E. Segall, Ph.D., Dept. of Physiology/Anatomy, UC, Berkeley; Benjamin S. Frank, M.D., leading voice in nucleic-acid therapy; Thomas Donaldson, Ph.D., associate editor of *Long Life Magazine*; Robert Prehoda, Ph.D., author of *Extended Youth*; Saul Kent, director of the Alcor Life Extension Conference and author of *The Life Extension Revolution*; Robert Parker, Ph.D., formerly of the Roche Institute of Molecular Biology; Constance Tsao, Ph.D., of the Pauling Institute of Science and Medicine; Ronald K. Siegel, Ph.D., of the UCLA School of Medicine; Thomas Kappeler, M.D.; Robert Anton Wilson, Ph.D., Senior Professor of Science and Humanities, Paideia University, San Francisco; Steven Fowkes, Jim Welch, Nat Hall, and Skye d'Aureous.

Finally, and most gratefully of all, I want to thank Janis for her patience and support during the writing and production of the book.

John Mann
The Megahealth Society
Box 1684  Manhattan Beach, CA 90266
June 24, 1980

# Chapter One

# The Life-Extension Story

*Many people who are reading this book may live for 200 years or more. Studies with laboratory animals show that we now have the essential medical technology to extend human lifespan from its present average of 75 years to somewhere between 100 and 120 years. Scientists believe that we may soon be able to go far beyond that. A number of "youth drugs" already exist, but medical politics prevents physicians from prescribing them. Nevertheless, they are freely available, and many people are using them on their own.*

*This condensed history gives an introductory, over-all picture of the material detailed in the rest of the book. It attempts to provide a background that will place in perspective the present theories of aging and the events that have brought the science of life extension to its present stage.*

The science of gerontology has had many false beginnings, often because of grandiose blunders. We can easily understand why they happened, when we consider how desperately men have searched for a way to stave off the inevitable decline of life. Legend and history are filled with tales of this search. The Sumerian hero-king, Gilgamesh, despondent over the death of his friend Enkidu, and seeing that his own days were also numbered, sought the herb of eternal life. He found it, only to have it eaten by a serpent while he slept. The aging sixteenth-century conquistador, Luis Ponce de Leon, searched the New World for the Fountain of Youth, but instead discovered what is now the world's most famous old folks' home: Florida.

Haunted by the brevity of earthly existence, humans have fabricated elaborate institutions to convince themselves that some sort of life continues after this one. Christians built cathedrals, and Pharaohs fashioned pyramids; yet they all bargained for the same thing. If eternal life could not be had on Earth, a compro-

"Why was I born if it wasn't forever?"

George Ionesco

"In almost any other important biological field than that of senescence, it is possible to present the main theories historically, and to show a steady progression from a large number of speculative, to one or two highly probable, main hypotheses. In the case of senescence, this cannot be profitably done. . . . It is a striking feature of these theories that they show little or no historical development; they can much more readily be summarized as a catalogue than as a process of developing scientific awareness."

Alex Comfort,
*Ageing: The Biology of Senescence*

mise might be made for immortality beyond the grave. Even with a theological guarantee of afterlife everlasting, men and women have remained easy prey for the peddler of dubious potions who promises a few additional years of life.

Few but dreamers and fools have expected that physical life might last for eternity. But the wise were often convinced that it need not be quite so fleeting. There have even been occasional instances of inordinate longevity to support their convictions. One of the more famous of these was Thomas Parr, an English peasant, who is reported to have lived for more than a century and a half, sustaining himself on a frugal diet of fruit, cheese, and black bread. In 1635, he was brought before the court of King Charles, where he was lavishly wined and dined by those who hoped to learn his secret. He soon died of overindulgence. William Harvey, the famed discoverer of the circulatory system, performed the autopsy, and declared that Parr's 152-year-old brain and organs were in a marvelous state of preservation.

Many people have lived well beyond the century mark. Some practiced moderation. Others indulged in noxious vices. Each claimed that his own lifestyle, wholesome or decadent, was the cause of his longevity. Those who sought a formula or set of rules for long life could find little consistency in the habits of centenarians. The best prerequisites seemed to be good genes and the will to survive.

## The Beginnings of Gerontology

Toward the end of the nineteenth century, man's knowledge of physiology had expanded some. Taken with their new awareness of the endocrine system, men of science began to view these glands and their secretions as possible keys to youth, vitality, and long life. In the spring of 1889, the 72-year-old physiologist Charles Edouard Brown-Sequard conducted rejuvenation experiments upon himself with injections of dog-testicle extracts. His results, in his own eyes, were remarkable. He felt thirty years younger, and even measured muscular improvements. But his colleagues and his young wife saw him as the senile fool and dupe of his own placebo. He died a few years later of a stroke.

Despite Brown-Sequard's unprofessional self-deception and humiliating downfall, many other scientists felt that his work had been pointing in a valid direction. Ironically, his attempt and failure stirred others into a more active search for the glandular key to rejuvenation. Many gerontologists now regard June 1, 1889, the date of Brown-Sequard's announcement of his experiment, as the birthdate of modern gerontology.[43]

Shortly after Brown-Sequard, the Viennese endocrinologist Eugen Steinach attempted rejuvenation by tying off the sperm ducts, supposedly to reroute the male sex hormones from the testes to the bloodstream. The results of his experiments with rats and humans seemed to substantiate his approach, but modern endocrinologists can find no reason why the operation should have had any physiological effect other than sterility. Essentially, Steinach's operation was the same vasoligature procedure used today for birth control. There have been a few sporadic reports of increased vitality after vasectomy, but most men who have undergone this surgery have experienced no such changes. Time and observation may eventually yield an explanation.

Steinach's contemporary, Serge Voronoff, catered to the wealthy with testicular grafts from young monkeys; his fees began at $5,000. His career began with apparent sincerity, grew corrupt with multimillion-dollar profits, and ended in disgrace and tragedy when his grafts failed to take and it was found that he had transferred syphilis from his monkeys to his patients.

Except for some outrageous charlatans—mostly in the United States—Steinach and Voronoff inspired no disciples. For the orthodox gerontologist, glandular transplants were a closed and unwelcome subject. An exception, perhaps, was Paul Niehans, a Swiss surgeon, who did not actually follow in the footsteps of Steinach and Voronoff, but rather learned from their mistakes. He developed a technique called cell therapy, which involves injection of fresh cells from the organs of a sheep fetus. The testimonials of numerous celebrities, including Pope Pius XII, gave credibility to Niehans' work. No one can explain why cell therapy works, and many professionals doubt that it does; yet today, six years after Niehans' death at 89, his famous clinic in Vevey still stands, and thousands every year are treated there.

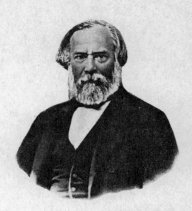

*Charles Edouard Brown-Sequard*
*1817–1894*

## Carrel's Cultures and the Hayflick Limit

Curiously, Niehans' inspiration for cell therapy came from another of gerontology's grandiose blunders, the erroneous discoveries of the French physiologist Alexis Carrel, who won the Nobel Prize for other, valid work.

In 1912, at the Rockefeller Institute, Carrel started a tissue culture of fibroblast cells from the heart of a chicken embryo, and replenished the culture medium regularly with a crude extract drawn from other chicken embryos. The culture grew proliferously, and far outlived control cultures that were maintained on ordinary nutrients. In fact, the culture was still alive in 1946, two years after Carrel's death, when his coworkers terminated the experiment.

From this study Carrel and others theorized that living cells, when isolated from their parent organism, are essentially immortal; that some factor in young or embryonic tissue can maintain youth and vigor, and ensure that immortality; and that this factor can be transferred as a nutrient from its source to other, older tissues.

"The basic purpose of all this business is: How do we get to live longer better? If we can't live longer, let's live better. I think we can do both, though."

Denham Harman,
quoted in *The Youth Doctors* by
Patrick McGrady, Jr.

Carrel's experiment caused a revolution in gerontology and general physiology. If the life-sustaining factor could be isolated and synthesized, humanity might have a cure for aging and an elixir of eternal life. Other researchers, however, were unable to duplicate Carrel's results. Little was heard at first about their failures, because they wanted neither to contradict what stood as established truth nor to admit the possibility of their own ineptness. Some workers conducted the experiment with cells of other animals, and many who tried it with the embryonic cells of mice had apparent success. This gave further support to Carrel's dogma, and deepened the self-doubts of those whose cultures did not survive.

During the 1960s, Leonard Hayflick and Paul Moorhead at the Wistar Institute in Philadelphia made a thorough study of the issue. They ultimately established that normal cells will divide a given number of times; this number is known as the Hayflick Limit. Cell divisions will slow down and cease as they reach this limit, and the culture will die. Carrel's culture, they realized, had survived because the embryonic extract added to the medium had been improperly prepared, and was often contaminated with live chick cells. [139] One of Carrel's assistants later admitted to Hayflick that she knew of this contamination, but dared not voice criticism. [308]

Hayflick's studies uncovered some other pertinent facts. It had been known that cancer cells are potentially immortal (they are also suicidal, in that they eventually destroy their host). In 1952, George O. Gey at Johns Hopkins University School of Medicine had excised cancerous cells from the cervix of a woman named Henrietta Lacks, and had cultured these in an ordinary nutrient medium. These now-famous HeLa cells proliferated, and portions of them have been sent to laboratories all over the world for further study. These and the parent culture still survive and will doubtlessly continue to do so. Hayflick found that mouse-embryo cells cultivated in a glass vessel spontaneously transform into abnormal cells that behave in many ways like cancer cells. When they are injected into animals, cancerous tumors develop. Furthermore, these cells, like cancer cells, are essentially immortal; that is, they will continue to divide and multiply indefinitely. This is why some workers could duplicate Carrel's results when mouse cells were substituted for chick cells. This phenomenon occurs frequently with mouse cells in an enclosed glass vessel, but only rarely with the cells of humans, chickens, or other animals. [140]

Almost fifty years had elapsed between the establishment of Carrel's dogma of cellular immortality and Hayflick's rectification of the error. During that half-century, many gerontological studies had been based on Carrel's spurious premises. One might think that all this research had been wasted; but that was not the case. Not since Brown-Sequard's illustrious failure had the science of gerontology known such a spurt of enthusiasm. Much research of this period, although inspired by false data, was fruitful and revealing. For one thing, Leonard Hayflick's work was largely an outgrowth of Carrel's mistake.

Hayflick discovered that normal human embryonic fibroblasts *in vitro* (cultured outside of the organism; literally, in glassware) will divide and replicate approximately 50 times before they perish. This takes about two years. The process, of course, is swifter *in vitro* than *in vivo* (in the living organism). This figure, 50 replications, plus or minus 10, is the Hayflick Limit. Older human cells and embryonic fibroblasts of shorter-lived species will replicate a correspondingly fewer number of times, and the durations of their cultures can be more or less predicted from the Hayflick Limit. With Hayflick's mathematics, one can also calculate the potential average maximum lifespan of any species from the number of times its embryonic cells will divide *in vitro*. Using this approach, Hayflick estimates that a human lifespan should be roughly 110 to 120 years.

This raises several questions. What is it that limits human cell cultures to 50 doublings, and human lifespan to 120 years? Why do so few humans ever attain this maximum? There have been some serious and worthwhile attempts to answer these questions, but none, so far, have explained everything satisfactorily. Some of these proposals conflict, at times, with others; but most of them connect as pieces in a large, unfinished puzzle.

## Free Radicals and Immune Deterioration

One lucidly connecting group of theories concerns the highly reactive molecular fragments known as free radicals, which are created in the metabolic system by several causes, including radiation and the uncontrolled oxidation of fats. These radicals readily attach themselves to other molecules of the body; often to the long, fibrous protein structures, and sometimes to the DNA and RNA within the cells. Whatever they link with, they alter both structurally and functionally. This theory was first put forth in 1941 by Johan Bjorksten, who had been working as a research chemist for Ditto, Inc. (a branch of Eastman Kodak). He had noticed the resemblance between the aging of film materials and that of the human body. He blamed the senescence of living organisms on the formation of cross-linking bridges between protein molecules, and also between strands of DNA or RNA, which then synthesize defective proteins. [20, 21]

In the early 1950s, Denham Harman at the University of Nebraska greatly increased the lifespan of mice by adding various antioxidants and free-radical deactivators to their diet. Other workers have had similar results with antioxidants, and some have reported even more spectacular results from using combinations

"And God said: My spirit shall not always dwell in man, since he is of flesh; yet the number of his days shall be one hundred and twenty years."

*Genesis* 6:3

"Such reshuffling of genetic information when egg and sperm cells are produced or fused could perhaps serve to reprogram or reset the cell's biological clock. By this mechanism, even if the individual members of a species were programmed to die, the species would live. A human being, then, would be the germ cell's way of making more immortal germ cells."

Leonard Hayflick

of these substances, which, it appears, may have mutually potentiating interactions.

The free-radical/cross-linkage proposition has several points of contact with other explanations of aging, including the immunological theory. It has long been established that our immunological defenses weaken with age, and that autoimmune diseases are more common in later years. In 1969 Roy Walford of UCLA[393] published a theory that attributes both phenomena to changes in the immune cells and antibodies that result from loss, alteration, or blurring of genetic information. Not only does the effectiveness of the immune system against foreign, disease-causing microorganisms dwindle with age, but our immune cells also lose their ability to make a clear distinction between native protein and foreign protein. Unable to tell friend from foe, the cells and antibodies frequently attack the body's own tissues and enzymes. To further confound the aging immune system, the cross-linked and misconstructed proteins are altered enough to appear genuinely foreign. There is also some evidence that certain slow-acting but persistent viruses bring about senile changes in the immune system by subtly altering the coding of the DNA. If this is so, aging may be truly regarded as a disease rather than as a normal phase of life.

Since the early 1930s, scientists have been able to delay maturation in animals and extend animal lifespans by restricting their caloric intake to a bare minimum.[223] Similar, though lesser, results have been achieved with protein restriction and diets deficient in the amino acid tryptophan. As far back as 1917, workers had lengthened the lives of cold-blooded animals by keeping their environment 6°C lower than normal. In recent years, similar results with warm-blooded animals have been achieved by manipulating the temperature-regulating mechanism in the brain. Temperature reduction (hypothermia) combined with caloric restriction has resulted in the greatest life extensions thus far. Roy Walford found that both hypothermia and dietary restriction suppress the immune system's activity and retard its decline. Safe and comfortable methods of lowering human body temperature are now being sought. Most researchers believe that a reduction of just a few degrees could double human lifespan.

## What Controls Aging?

Despite the collapse of Carrelian theory, the suspicion has persisted that there may be a youth factor in young or embryonic tissues that can rejuvenate older tissues. This suspicion led to experiments with parabiosis, the joining together of the circulatory systems of an old creature and a young creature of the same species. The results were partial rejuvenation of the older animals, [163, 164, 314] and, in some respects, accelerated aging of the younger ones. [297, 380] This suggests that senescence may be caused not only by the depletion of a youth factor, but also by the presence of an aging factor, which either accumulates over the years or is produced or released at a particular time in the organism's life cycle. There are some clues to what this substance is, where it comes from, and how it operates, but more answers are needed.

The major question, however, that gerontologists have been asking is whether the primary causes of aging are central or cellular. Does a mechanism in one of the body's control centers—the endocrines, the nervous system, the brain—initiate the release of some hormonal substance that signals the cells to cease operations, or is each cell programmed from birth to turn off at a particular time?

Hayflick's experiments suggest that aging is entirely a cellular response. If cells have a given maximum lifespan when cultured *in vitro*, why suspect any organ or secretion as the culprit? Still, there are many who do, and who have experimental evidence that some mechanism in the hypothalamus and pituitary signals the cells to age and die. The neurohormone serotonin has been implicated as one of the substances involved in triggering the release of a "death hormone." Some gerontologists believe that other glands, such as the thymus and thyroid, are the initiators of aging. It is likely that all these organs are in some ways involved.

Researchers who think that aging is generated in the cells are divided on whether the process takes place in the cytoplasm or in the nucleus. Many hold that senescence first occurs in the mitochondria, the tiny organelles that populate the cell's cytoplasmic ocean and carry out the body's energy transformations. Others accuse another organelle, the scavenging lysosome, of rupturing and polluting the cytoplasm with its load of toxic wastes. Two researchers at New York State University in Buffalo caused a virtually immortal species of amoeba to age rapidly and die by transferring to it cytoplasmic material from a short-lived species. [237] This could demonstrate that the cellular cause of aging resides in the cytoplasm rather than the nucleus. But when Hayflick separated the nuclei from the cytoplasm of human cells and recombined the young nuclei with cells containing old cytoplasm, and vice versa, it was always the age of the nucleus, not that of the cytoplasm, which determined how many doublings remained before the cells reached the Hayflick Limit. A contradiction, perhaps; but it may be that the aging mechanism of amoebas and other one-celled life forms differs from that of complex organisms.

If the aging mechanism of the cell resides within the nucleus, the fault may be in the DNA molecule, the coded blueprint of life itself. The big riddle, then, is how this mechanism

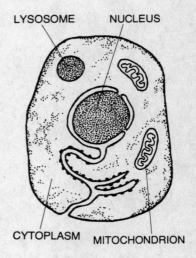

*Simplified animal cell.*

"The consensus at the moment appears to be that aging represents the loss of biological information."

Alex Comfort,
*Geriatrics*, (March 1970)

works. It could be that the DNA, with all of its programmed hereditary data, contains a genetic order to age at a given rate over the years and to self-destruct at an approximate time. Or it may be that the DNA's fundamental message—to live, to multiply, to survive—becomes blurred and distorted with time and replication, until this message is lost. Perhaps DNA replication is like photocopying. A copy of a copy of a copy, and so on, would lose more and more of its original clarity with each duplication, until its contents are scarcely legible.

Several hypotheses propose that aging results from somatic mutations, that is, coding changes in the DNA of the body's dividing cells (as opposed to genetic mutations, which occur in reproductive cells). Zhores A. Medvedev, of the National Institute for Medical Research in London, believes that aging stems from accumulation of errors in the DNA and RNA. He suggests that the control of the programming and expression of the genes is the key to the prevention of aging.[228] Leslie Orgel, of the Salk Institute at La Jolla, holds that random errors in the synthesis of protein structures occur frequently. Those in minor, nonvital structures can be corrected by the cell, but those in the protein portions of the enzymes that carry out protein synthesis are irreversible and cumulative. As these errors increase in number, aging and gradual death take place.[250]

Critics of these theories point out that each cell contains genes for every organ and tissue of the body; since only the genes that pertain to a cell's particular role are expressed, somatic mutations of any significance would therefore be very rare. Also, these theories do not account for aging in creatures like the fruit fly, whose cells cease division at maturity.[319]

Gerontologists are also considering the possibility that the cerebral centers of the brain may influence aging. The neural cells of the brain do not divide and replicate. When they die, they are not replaced. Also, the efficiency of many living brain cells is impaired because of age pigment, amyloid deposits, cross-links, and reduced supplies of oxygen and nourishment. It has been proposed that one function of the collective of brain cells is to preside over the vital cellular activities which perpetuate the conditions of youth. When brain-cell efficiency and number are reduced, youth fades and aging takes place.[360] There are facts and findings to support this thesis. For one thing, Mongoloids and other mentally retarded persons tend to age prematurely.[90]

Since the time of Brown-Sequard's self-injection of dog-testicle extracts, endocrinology has come a long way. It is now realized that the self-deceived "father" of gerontology was on the right track, but in the wrong train. Although hormonal failures are responsible for losses of vitality and good appearance during aging, and although injections of certain steroid hormones can improve these conditions, such injections do not now seem to be

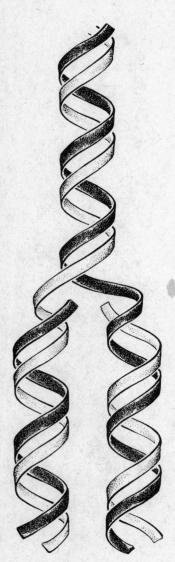

*DNA duplicating.*

a way to extend lifespan substantially. The endocrine problem in aging is that there is a decrease not only in hormone production, but also in the body's ability to use its hormones. [108, 317, 318, 385] Once science and medicine have learned how to correct the senile loss of receptivity to these secretions, the way may be open to study the effectiveness of hormone supplementation in extending human lifespan.

Catecholamines are another class of hormones, involved in nerve-impulse transmission, brain activity, energy levels, and mood. These also undergo changes during aging, changes that are responsible for many of the discomforts of the aged, and that may contribute to the deterioration process itself. The catecholamines include such substances as norepinephrine and dopamine. Both the amounts of these brain amines that are present and the body's receptivity to their actions diminish with age. The main antiaging function of the controversial Romanian procaine compound Gerovital H3, which we will discuss later, is that it prevents destruction of certain essential catecholamines that tend to dwindle in later life.

Improper nutrition is known to hasten aging, and increased daily intake of some vitamins and minerals has extended the lifespans of laboratory animals. The modern psychiatric technique of megavitamin therapy, which recognizes that certain individuals require larger than normal amounts of some nutrients for sound mental functioning, has its counterpart in modern gerontology. Several herbs, including ginseng, have also been found to slow the rate of aging to some extent, and to improve health and vitality in aging persons.

The theories and hypotheses about aging discussed so far are not the only ones with merit. Several others concerning general wear and tear on various components of the body, [38] increments of stresses which deplete a limited reservoir of adaptive energy, and the accumulation of toxic metabolic wastes in the cells and tissues [333] also deserve further investigation.

## Combatting the Effects of Aging

No single factor can be pinpointed as *the* cause of aging. Each contributes in its own way to hastening our decline and departure. As in warfare, although just one of the attacker's several forces — its artillery, its air power, its infantry — may cinch the conquest, all were in their own manners responsible for predisposing the victim to the final blow.

Gerontologists not only look for causes of aging, but also try to learn how known causes interact to augment each other's effects. The late Howard J. Curtis of the Brookhaven National Laboratory described in his *composite theory of aging* how such factors as radiation, mutation, and toxic accumulations mutually

"The people proposing aging theories remind me somewhat of the story of the seven blind men examining an elephant: to the one feeling a leg, an elephant is like a tree; the one feeling the trunk thought he was like a big snake, etc.; each being correct so far as he went. So with the aging theories, each is probably correct to a certain extent."

Denham Harman, quoted in *Extended Youth* by Robert Prehoda

"What really troubles the organism is the increasing disharmony of mutual relations among the various component activities — a loss of integration."

Paul Weiss,
in *Perspectives in Experimental Gerontology*

"Today, if you can buy 50 years, you may look forward to eternity."

Arthur Quaife,
ALCOR Conference

influence one another to increase the rate of physical degeneration.[53] In their *integrated theory of aging*, Carpenter and Loynd explain how interactions of stress, metabolic waste production, free-radical buildup, and somatic mutations work together to accelerate the rate of cross-linkage and other molecular changes that immobilize many of the body's active molecules.[38] Similarly, in the *combination theory of aging*, Hans Kugler shows how several primary causes of aging form "aging initiators," while secondary causes (stress factors that the body could have coped with one at a time, but which are overwhelming in combination) accelerate the rate of aging.[197]

Without pursuing the details of these theories, we can see that destructive elements are more damaging when they occur in combination. Conversely, it is reasonable to assume that any therapies that resist interrelated causes of aging will be more effective when jointly applied. Richard Passwater, of the American Instrument Company in Silver Spring, Maryland, combined antioxidants and extended the lives of test animals by as much as 67 per cent. Previous extensions with single antioxidants ranged between 20 and 50 per cent.[188, 204]

The next step in studying the synergistic relationships of life-extension techniques is to combine therapies that combat different contributing causes of aging; that is, not only antioxidants and free-radical deactivators, but also optimal nutrition, megadosages of certain vitamins, serotonin normalizers, protein-synthesis enhancers, DNA repair aids, and other treatments described in this book. Although we know of no animal experiments in which this is being done, there are thousands of humans who have been self-experimenting for years with these combined therapies. It will take many more years to find out just what effect these measures have had on their longevity, but so far these persons report great improvements in health, vitality, and appearance.

It is because of idiosyncrasies in the medical and governmental control of new pharmaceuticals that most of these life-extension drugs can be obtained easily and inexpensively. For ethical and practical reasons, scientific experiments with these drugs are initially conducted with short-lived animals. Though it takes only two or three years to demonstrate that a drug will extend the normal 18- to 24-month lifespan of a rodent by 50 per cent, it would require about a century to prove conclusively that it can do the same for a human. The biological mechanisms by which these longevity drugs operate, however, are common to all mammals, and there is little or no doubt that they can also slow down the aging rate in humans. Most of these materials have been shown to be safe — and often immediately beneficial — when used properly. Still, the medical profession and the Food and Drug Administration cannot permit the drugs to be sold or prescribed as pharmaceuticals until all the final proofs of effectiveness in humans have been given. Unfortunately, by that time most of us will be too old to benefit from them.

When these substances have been found to be effective as antiaging drugs for humans, they will undoubtedly be classified as prescription-only items and sold at the usual exorbitant drug-company prices. Until that time, though, they have no officially recognized pharmaceutical value, and are therefore sold inexpensively as ordinary chemicals. This situation has been a blessing for the many self-experimenting longevists who have been using life-extension drugs on their own. These longevists are generally aware of the "unproven" status of the drugs, but are satisfied by the existing data that the drugs are safe and efficacious; and if they wait for the usual medical and governmental sanctions, they will have missed this opportunity for prolonged youth and extended lifespan.

What makes this pursuit of longevity most enticing is that there may be much more at stake than extensions of a mere 30 or 40 years. Leading gerontologists believe that with the proper funding they can find ways to double human lifespan within the next 10 to 20 years. The success of such therapies would largely depend on a person's physical state when treatments are commenced. By the time such life-extension methods are developed and approved for clinical testing on volunteers, all of us will be at least 20 or 30 years older. By using presently known antiaging therapies, however, a person may maintain a biological age that is far younger than his chronological one. If, for example, a person is 30 now, and life-doubling therapies become available when he is 60, they are likely to be of only limited value for him. But if he has been following a longevity program with the existing therapies described in this book, his biological age may be only 40 or 45 at that time. By so minimizing and delaying the senile degeneration of his body, he may still be eligible for an even greater extension of lifespan. When the more effective therapies are available, he may gain an additional century in which to hope for another gerontological breakthrough that could offer him a lifespan of 300, 400, or even 500 years. In that much time, science may even find the key to immortality.

For those of us who desire long life, this is an attractive prospect. At worst we can improve our health and add a few years to life. At best we may become candidates for a series of extensions that would ultimately stretch the days of our lives far beyond the number allegedly enjoyed by Methuselah. Some among us may not wish to linger that long on Earth. There are many who feel that the average allotment of three score years and ten is cross enough to bear in this world. But there are many others who love being alive, and who believe that even the longest lifespan that humans have come to expect—90 to 100 years—is too pre-

"Try to stay alive a little longer."

Robert C. W. Ettinger,
*The Prospect of Immortality*

"Some people want to achieve immortality through their works or their descendants. I prefer to achieve immortality by not dying."

Woody Allen

ciously brief for us to fulfill even a fraction of our possibilities and aspirations. As one of our Megahealth Society members has rather anachronistically declared, "We want immortality, and we want it now!"

But does anything that even approaches immortality fall within the realm of possibility? Or are there limiting factors that would prevent us under any circumstances from living beyond a given age?

Since the debunking of Alexis Carrel's famed chick-embryo experiment and the almost universal acceptance of the Hayflick Limit, it has seemed that the maximum degrees of life extension are fixed by the mortal nature of the living cell. Recently, however, Hayflick's theories have begun to show their age. A number of findings indicate that Carrel's faultily conducted experiment might have borne out his cherished beliefs if this otherwise great scientist had not been so eager to prove himself correct. More recent tissue-culture experiments, described in the commitment theory of Holliday and Tarrant,[159] have begun to dispel the terrible implication of finality in the Hayflick Limit, and hint that under the right conditions our cells may be potentially immortal. This does not mean that Hayflick's contributions are invalid. The Hayflick Limit consistently reflects the probable lifespan of a creature, and is a useful tool for conducting preliminary *in vitro* studies of new life-extension therapies. Revisions of theories are to be expected in an infant science still struggling to establish its foundations.

# Chapter Two

# Stopping Chemical Damage Within

## Free Radicals and Cross-Linkage

*Antioxidants are the largest and most frequently used group of life-extension drugs. They interfere with certain harmful reactions within the body that create extensive damage: body proteins become cross-linked and tangled; the tissues lose their suppleness; the arteries harden and are more likely to collect cholesterol; susceptibility to cancer increases; and the genetic information needed to regenerate the body becomes distorted. These are only the beginning of a long sequence of things that go wrong.*

*Most of the famous life-extension experiments in laboratory animals have been done with antioxidants. They are also among the least expensive and most accessible longevity drugs.*

A free radical is a portion of a molecule that has become separated during a chemical reaction. Because free radicals carry one or more unpaired electrons, they are usually highly reactive. They will attempt to unite with almost any other molecule they come in contact with, but they do unite more readily with certain molecules than with others. When they react and combine with the long molecules of fibrous protein, these proteins become cross-linked, or bound together at their middles. If this biochemical handcuffing happens enough, the normal functions of these proteins are hampered.

Cross-linkage binds various types of fibrous protein, including the collagen, elastin, and reticulin of the connective tissue. Collagen makes up about a fourth of the body's protein. It is often called the mortar of the cells. Collagen structurally supports the living cells of the body. Moisture, oxygen, and nourishment must travel through the collagen to reach the cells, and it is also through the network of collagen that waste products are transferred to the avenues of excretion.

"Man is as old as his connective tissues."
Alexandr Bogomolets

13

"The effect [cross-linking] is like what would happen in a large factory with thousands of workers if someone slipped a pair of handcuffs on one hand of each of two workers, to tie them together. This obviously would reduce their ability to do their work, and if the process were allowed to spread through the factory, even at a slow rate, it would ultimately paralyze the entire operation unless means were found to remove the handcuffs faster than they were being applied."

Johan Bjorksten

"The human body dies only because we have forgotten how to transform it and change it."

Antonin Artaud, *Theater and Science*

The condition of the collagen and other connective tissues can make the skin look smooth or wrinkled, saggy or resilient; the eyes clear or cloudy; the carriage erect or stooped. When the body is in its infant stage, the connective tissue has a pliable, almost jelly-like, quality. At that time, most of this tissue consists of a soft material called ground substance. As time passes, the connective tissue becomes tougher and firmer. This change is due to cross-linkage. During growth, much of the ground substance is converted to collagen, and the collagen molecules, in turn, become bound to one another by means of chemical reactions. The same thing happens to leather during the tanning process: its molecules become cross-linked, and it becomes tougher and less resilient.

It is normal and healthy for this cross-linking process to take place during our earliest years. If it didn't, our bodies would remain as delicate and vulnerable as those of babies. The problem is that the process does not stop when we have reached adulthood. Instead, it continues at an increasing rate, and the collagen tightens and shrinks so much that it strangles the cells, constricts the tiny capillaries, and chokes off the supply of blood, with its cargo of oxygen, moisture, and nourishment. As this happens, the skin becomes leathery and wrinkled, the arteries lose their ability to expand and contract, the joints and cartilage stiffen, and every part of the body gradually deteriorates. Toxic waste products accumulate in the cells and contribute further to the body's ruin.

During youth, the body produces enzymes that break down excessive cross-linkages almost as swiftly as they occur. Between the cross-linking substances and the unlinking enzymes, we have a balance of power that keeps the tissues firm but elastic. But as we grow older, the cross-linking reactions take place faster than these enzymes can undo them, because there is a gradual reduction in the production of the enzymes and a continuing accumulation of cross-linking substances.

Aside from natural agents that the body produces to cross-link a percentage of our infant collagen, there are many external sources of free radicals or of agents that generate them. These include pollutants, cigarette smoke, polyvalent metals (lead, cadmium, etc.), sodium nitrite (a cold-cut preservative), aldehydes, dibasic acids, nitrogen oxides, sulfur dioxides, ozone, radiation (X-rays, cosmic radiation, nuclear by-products, fallout, etc.), and some foods, especially those which are rancid or lacking in freshness. Another source of cross-linking agents is toxic residues from exhaustion, illness, and stress.

Free radicals can be normal products of the body's metabolic processes. Many are involved in biochemical reactions that are essential to life. These are usually controlled by enzymes, and produce smooth, harmless reactions. But formation of too many of these violently reacting free radicals results in protein cross-linkage and hastens aging.

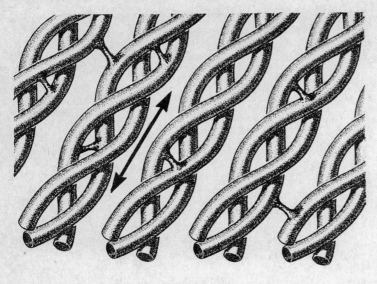

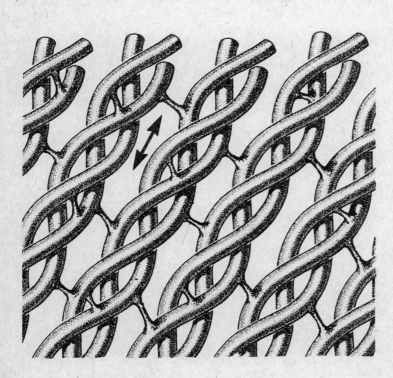

*Collagen and cross-linking of collagen.*

This model of collagen shows the remarkable architecture of connective tissue. Each of the tube structures represents a chain of amino acids. Three such chains twisted together in a spiral (a triple helix) are considered a unit of collagen. Many of these units are joined end to end to form long, continuous threads; in turn, these continuous threads are stacked side by side to form larger strands. A small section of one of those strands is shown here.

During youth, there is a moderate amount of cross-linking to tie the collagen threads to each other (shown in the top half of the picture). As a result, the collagen threads slide past each other, and the connective tissue is quite elastic. With increasing age, more cross-links are formed; these tie more collagen threads to each other, and the sliding of threads past each other becomes greatly restricted (shown in the bottom half of the picture). The result is less-elastic connective tissue.

*Initiation:* energy breaks a chemical bond, leaving one unpaired electron on each resulting piece.

Energy such as light, radioactivity, x-rays, etc.

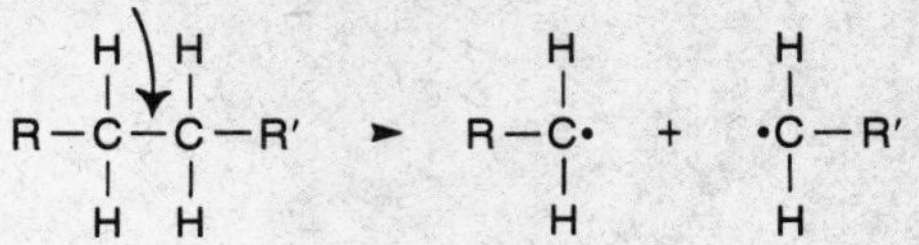

$$R-\overset{\overset{\displaystyle H}{|}}{\underset{\underset{\displaystyle H}{|}}{C}}-\overset{\overset{\displaystyle H}{|}}{\underset{\underset{\displaystyle H}{|}}{C}}-R' \;\blacktriangleright\; R-\overset{\overset{\displaystyle H}{|}}{\underset{\underset{\displaystyle H}{|}}{C}}\cdot \;+\; \cdot\overset{\overset{\displaystyle H}{|}}{\underset{\underset{\displaystyle H}{|}}{C}}-R'$$

*Propagation:* many types of reactions occur; a cross-linking reaction is shown here.

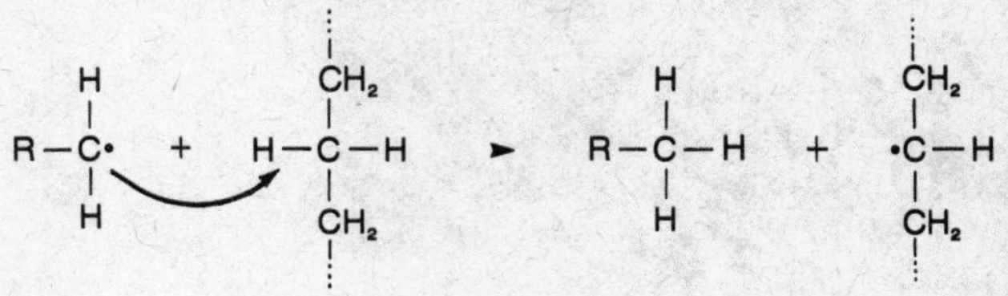

$$R-\overset{\overset{\displaystyle H}{|}}{\underset{\underset{\displaystyle H}{|}}{C}}\cdot \;+\; H-\overset{\overset{\displaystyle CH_2}{|}}{\underset{\underset{\displaystyle CH_2}{|}}{C}}-H \;\blacktriangleright\; R-\overset{\overset{\displaystyle H}{|}}{\underset{\underset{\displaystyle H}{|}}{C}}-H \;+\; \cdot\overset{\overset{\displaystyle CH_2}{|}}{\underset{\underset{\displaystyle CH_2}{|}}{C}}-H$$

The free radical attacks a bond in a long molecule, removes a hydrogen, and creates a free radical on the long molecule. This new free radical could attack another long molecule, forming a cross-link and creating an H· radical, as we see below.

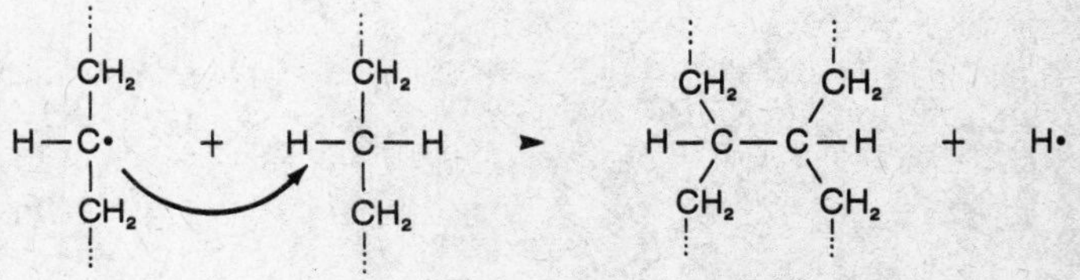

$$H-\overset{\overset{\displaystyle CH_2}{|}}{\underset{\underset{\displaystyle CH_2}{|}}{C}}\cdot \;+\; H-\overset{\overset{\displaystyle CH_2}{|}}{\underset{\underset{\displaystyle CH_2}{|}}{C}}-H \;\blacktriangleright\; H-\overset{\overset{\displaystyle CH_2}{|}}{\underset{\underset{\displaystyle CH_2}{|}}{C}}-\overset{\overset{\displaystyle CH_2}{|}}{\underset{\underset{\displaystyle CH_2}{|}}{C}}-H \;+\; H\cdot$$

*A more complicated type of cross-linking occurs when the long molecules are polyunsaturated fatty acids, and oxygen is present. The resulting long-chain reaction ties large numbers of fatty acids together into polymers. This is great for hardening oil-based paints, but is hard on biological membranes.*

*Termination:* again, many types of reactions serve as terminators. A simple type is shown here.

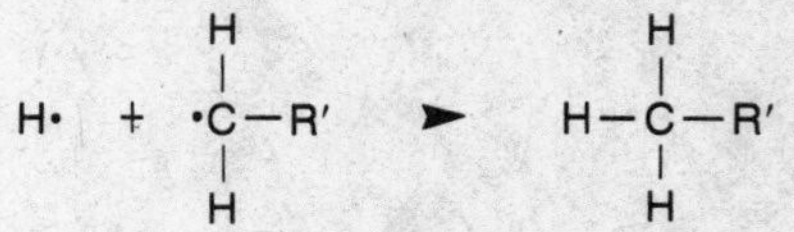

$$H\cdot \;+\; \cdot\overset{\overset{\displaystyle H}{|}}{\underset{\underset{\displaystyle H}{|}}{C}}-R' \;\blacktriangleright\; H-\overset{\overset{\displaystyle H}{|}}{\underset{\underset{\displaystyle H}{|}}{C}}-R'$$

*How free radicals can produce cross-linking.*

Two free radicals meet and combine their unpaired electrons into a stable chemical bond.

One of the major sources of harmful free radicals is a process known as lipid peroxidation. Lipids are a class of substances that include fats and oils. They are found throughout the body, stored in the tissues, at large in the bloodstream, molecularly joined to certain proteins (lipoproteins) and steroids, and involved in the structure of cell membranes and organelles. We derive many of these lipids from our foods as saturated and unsaturated fatty acids.

The unsaturated lipids react rapidly with oxygen from the atmosphere to form peroxides. This is what happens when fats and oils go rancid. It is a continuous process that begins the moment they are exposed to oxygen. We generally speak of a fat or oil as being rancid when the acrid odor and taste of rancidity has become overwhelming. But even in the freshest materials, the process of rancidification has already begun, nor does it cease after we have consumed the product. Lipids, stored in the tissues and circulating in the bloodstream, continue to combine with oxygen in the body, forming more peroxides and free radicals. To make matters worse, these highly unstable radicals, after being formed, link again with lipids and other bodily substances to form more such products in a continuing chemical chain reaction.

In order to control the aging process on this level, we must (1) prevent peroxidation of our foods during shipping and storage, (2) inhibit peroxidation of lipids in our bodies, (3) avoid or combat the causes of free-radical formation and cross-linkage (stress, toxins, radiation, etc.), (4) prevent free radicals from reacting with the body's proteins, by deactivating them before they can do harm, and (5) find enzymes or other agents that can safely break the cross-linking bonds and undo or correct other free-radical damage. [22, 130, 132, 133, 298, 299]

# Free-Radical Damage Within the Cells

The cell is the smallest unit within the body that can act alone, or interact with other cells, to perform all the fundamental functions of life. It is surrounded by a protective membrane. Inside this membrane is a more or less fluid substance called cytoplasm, which, like an ocean full of creatures, contains various subcellular bodies. Among these are several types of lipoprotein complexes, known as chondriosomes or organelles, which function in cell metabolism and secretion. These include: mitochondria, which are involved in all energy transformations within the cell; microsomes, which are essential to protein synthesis; and lysosomes, the tiny scavenger sacks that keep the intracellular environment clean by picking up the waste products of metabolism.

Each of these subcellular bodies is enveloped in its own protective membrane. Lipid peroxidation in these membranes can weaken and possibly rupture them. If this happens, the contents of the organelle may leak out and pollute the environment in the cell. The microsomes and mitochondria may contain complexly integrated enzyme systems, which, if they come in contact with peroxidized lipids and free radicals, can cause reactions which may seriously disrupt biochemical functions within the cell. If the lysosome membrane is broken, it will spill its load of waste products into the cytoplasm and release acid hydrolases, which do additional damage by autolysis (self-digestion) of the tissues. This is why lysosomes are often called the suicide bags of the cell. Some gerontologists believe that lysosome leakage may be one of the contributing causes of aging.[315] Some antiaging drugs can stabilize the lysosome membrane and prevent this sort of damage.

In the center of the cell is the nucleus. Here cell reproduction takes place. Every hereditary detail is coded in the DNA (deoxyribonucleic acid) molecules contained in the chromosomes of the nucleus. The RNA (ribonucleic acid) molecules in the cytoplasm act as messengers receiving instructions from the DNA to obtain the correct amino acids for protein synthesis. When products of lipid peroxidation react with DNA and RNA molecules and distort the genetic message, the proteins that are constructed are aberrant. If the body's immunological defense system no longer recognizes these proteins, it attacks them as it would any foreign proteins, bacteria, or viruses. The body then becomes its own enemy. Since enzymes are constructed of proteins, they too are affected. When the body is not producing enough properly formed enzymes, their necessary biochemical functions do not get performed; and an endless number of malfunctions can ensue. DNA and RNA distortions and the resulting protein missyntheses are now believed to play a significant role in the aging process.[195, 197] To deal with the problem, we must prevent the initial damage with antioxidants and free-radical deactivators, and assist the repair of the DNA or RNA molecule.

## Antioxidants and Free-Radical Deactivators

Antioxidants are substances that slow down the dangerous peroxidation of lipids, usually by presenting themselves as sacrificial material to be oxidized and thus use up the oxygen before it can react with the lipids. The products of such reactions are relatively stable and harmless compounds, which the body has little trouble metabolizing and eliminating. Free-radical deactivators — sometimes called free-radical scavengers — operate on a similar principle, reacting harmlessly with free radicals before these can react dangerously with vital components of the body. Most often, a substance that prevents peroxidation will also deactivate free radicals.

"Auto-oxidation appears to play a key role in aging. Experiments have shown a striking increase in the longevity of laboratory animals whose diet was supplemented with antioxidants such as BHT (a food preservative). The natural antioxidant vitamin E also seems to be important in the maintenance of cell function. There appears to be little reason to doubt that the judicious use and development of dietary supplements will add significantly to healthy life expectancy."

Bernard Strehler,
Santa Barbara Gerontology
Conference (1969)

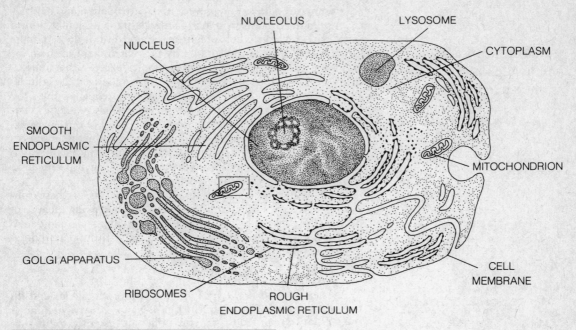

NUCLEOLUS

LYSOSOME

NUCLEUS

CYTOPLASM

SMOOTH ENDOPLASMIC RETICULUM

MITOCHONDRION

GOLGI APPARATUS

CELL MEMBRANE

RIBOSOMES

ROUGH ENDOPLASMIC RETICULUM

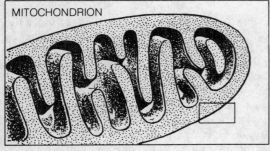

MITOCHONDRION

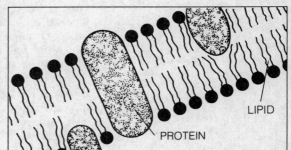

LIPID

PROTEIN

*Schematic of a typical human cell.*

Organelles are not drawn to exact scale here, to allow characteristic features to be illustrated. The membrane is a basic feature of every organelle in the cell. The location of the outer membrane of a mitochondrion is shown in this sequence of blow-ups; the picture would be similar for any of the other organelles or the cell membrane. Variations in composition exist, but the double lipid layer is a common feature. The heads (dark spot) of the lipid molecules have a high attraction for water and face outward; the tails (zig-zag line) of the lipid molecules, which prefer an oily environment, face each other. This creates an oily layer inside the membrane. The tails of these lipid molecules are the target of lipid peroxidation, especially if the lipids are polyunsaturated. Vitamin E normally works inside the membrane to prevent peroxidation, but if the lipid is unprotected, free radicals and oxygen can cause a chain reaction which polymerizes (ties together) these lipids and disrupts the membrane. This would then impair the function of the organelle and possibly damage the cell (as a broken lysosome would, for example).

"Health consists of
having the same diseases
as one's neighbors."

Quentin Crisp,
*The Naked Civil Servant*

*Ascorbic acid*

H
|
H—C—OH
|
HO—C—H
|
H

HO        OH

—2H        +2H

H
|
H—C—OH
|
HO—C—H
|
H

*Dehydroascorbic acid*

Some substances that prevent lipid peroxidation and neutralize free radicals are nutritional elements (trace minerals, amino acids, vitamins, and their precursors) found in our diets. Unfortunately, nature does not ordinarily provide enough of these for them to extend our lives to any measurable degree. Other antioxidants and free-radical deactivators are synthesized chemicals. These man-made molecules are often more effective than the natural ones. In a sense, they may be regarded as synthetic "vitamins" that have been missing from our diets all of our "natural" lives. A balanced combination of natural and synthetic substances appears to achieve the most outstanding results, mainly because these agents work synergistically, each doing its own specific task, while potentiating the others' effects.

We will now consider all pertinent aspects of these substances. We pay particular attention to ascorbic acid, because of its extraordinary role in health and longevity, and in order to resolve some of the controversial issues and misunderstandings that surround it.

## NATURAL ANTIOXIDANTS

*Ascorbic Acid (Vitamin C).*        Preventing colds and flu isn't all vitamin C is good for. In fact, it is more than a vitamin. It is a substance required in large quantities and essential to life, like water and oxygen.

Without ascorbic acid, human and animal life cannot exist. Most animals synthesize their own vitamin C in the liver or the kidneys. Human beings, other primates, and guinea pigs are among the few creatures that do not make their own, and must depend on outside sources. When a person is totally deprived of this vitamin, he develops scurvy. If this condition is allowed to persist, he will die a miserable death. It takes very little vitamin C to prevent scurvy. The National Research Council of the National Academy of Sciences bases the RDA (Recommended Daily Allowance) of ascorbic acid on the amount needed to prevent scurvy. However, this amount does not in any way indicate our actual requirements. The idea that we need only enough of the various vitamins, minerals, and other nutritional components to prevent the most obvious symptoms of deficiency — which is the current attitude of the medical establishment — contributes greatly toward keeping the general public at a mere subsistence level of health.

At this time, the RDA for vitamin C is 60 mg. For an average 150-pound human, this amount represents a little less than one milligram per kilogram of body weight. It is inconsistent that the Nutrient Requirements of Laboratory Animals from the Committee on Animal Nutrition recommends 55 mg per kilogram of body weight for monkeys.[45] Proportionally, for a 150-pound human, this would equal about 3,850 mg. In its native habitat, an adult gorilla will normally consume at least 4,500 mg of vitamin C daily in its diet of tropical fruits. Animals that synthesize their own ascorbic acid ordinarily produce about 70 mg per kilogram of body weight each day. If humans could manufacture their own vitamin C, a 150-pound person would therefore probably produce at least 5,000 mg daily, and this amount is probably closer to our actual needs. Under stress, an animal will produce more than three times the normal amount of this vitamin. Since twentieth-century man is under constant stress, and since environmental pollution destroys vitamin C in our bodies, the 150-pound human probably needs more than 15,000 mg of vitamin C daily. [364]

Until recently, the attitude of most scientists and nutritionists has been that if there was no scurvy, we were getting enough vitamin C. The absurdity in this reasoning is that scurvy is not the initial symptom of ascorbic-acid deficiency. It is the final stage preceding death. Enlightened physicians and nutritionists now use the term *subclinical scurvy* to indicate states in which we are getting enough of the vitamin to avoid symptoms of acute and chronic scurvy, but not enough to prevent less dramatic disorders.

A few milligrams of ascorbic acid daily will prevent acute scurvy. But when stress is placed on this short supply, symptoms of chronic scurvy may appear. These may include bleeding gums, mental sluggishness, irritability, and borderline anemia. A few more milligrams can prevent these problems, but resistance to infections will still be low. Flu and colds will be frequent; illness will be prolonged, and recovery slow. The flesh will bruise easily, and injuries will heal slowly. Skin condition and muscle tone may be poor. Kidney and bladder stones may develop. [369] One may be susceptible to allergies. Signs of aging will occur earlier than they would if supplies of the vitamin were adequate.

When daily dosages of ascorbic acid are maintained in the thousands of milligrams, these susceptibilities usually cease. [368] A person will then rarely (if ever) contract a cold, the flu, or any bacterial or viral disorder. [260, 261, 365] Infections and injuries will heal rapidly, and bruises will be mild, occurring only after the most severe blows. [372] Dosages in the tens of thousands of milligrams can have even more profound results. Cancers and tumors may be prevented or regressed, [262, 365] and lifespan may be prolonged considerably. Wrinkling and other visible signs of aging will be delayed. [368] Mental senility, loss of sexual potency, stooped stature, arthritic pains, [367] and other misfortunes of aging will be warded off or entirely avoided, and youthful vigor will be prolonged. [368] Fragile, porous bones that fail to mend if broken are one of the greatest threats to the aged. If ascorbic-acid levels are high and other nutritional and hormonal factors are in order, mending will be almost as rapid at 80 or even 120, as it was at 40. [67, 68, 371, 372]

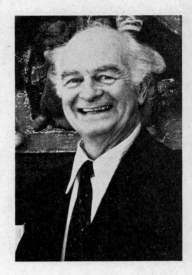

Linus Pauling, twice a Nobel laureate and recently a major proponent of the beneficial effects of large doses of ascorbic acid.

"Death is unnatural. . . . Theoretically, man is quite immortal."

Dr. Linus Pauling

Is vitamin C a cure-all, the ultimate wonder drug? It almost seems so, but only because of our past indoctrination. Our concept of good health has been so low that we have come to accept certain conditions as our lot in life. Now, people are beginning to see that ascorbic acid is not merely a vitamin, needed in traces, but an essential substance, required in plentiful amounts to maintain life and optimum health. The functions of ascorbic acid are so numerous that a deficiency will affect every organ and tissue of the body, and may result in a host of ailments. When ascorbic acid is properly supplied, these disorders disappear; so it appears to be a cure-all. Modern nutritionists prefer to regard ascorbic acid as a substance which was once—in our evolutionary history—our birthright, but which we were denied because a genetic mutation, which took place eons ago, made us unable to manufacture an enzyme required to synthesize this vital substance from glucose. When mankind migrated from areas where fruits rich in ascorbic acid were available all year round, and set up the patterns of living and eating that we know today, this substance dwindled in our diets. Not until the wheel had turned full circle, in the middle of this century, when we had isolated, synthesized, and understood the significance of this chemical, did it begin to come back into our lives on a scale that could meet our real needs.

It may seem a disadvantage that we must depend on external sources of ascorbic acid. But actually we are thus spared the burden of producing our own.[260] Also, when large amounts are needed to meet an emergency, we can take a large dose faster than, as animals, we could manufacture it.

Vitamin C's functions in health and the control of aging may be viewed in two categories: (a) everyday functions of fundamental dosages that meet our regular needs; (b) special functions, in which extra dosages are taken to cope with unusual situations of stress, disease, or poisoning. Unfortunately, in our hectic and polluted world, many of these "special" situations occur daily.

Among its everyday functions, ascorbic acid is essential in the synthesis of healthy protein, the formation and maintenance of collagen and other connective tissues, and the assimilation of calcium, iron, and other minerals. It integrates the spinal discs, helps to regulate cholesterol levels, and is involved in the formation of some enzymes and hormones. It concentrates in the optic lens, where it helps to maintain normal vision; is used by antibodies to destroy dangerous bacteria and viruses; and combines with toxins and wastes in the body, neutralizing them and rendering them soluble for excretion. It prevents fatigue by reducing acetone bodies left over when fats are burned for energy. It increases the efficiency of other nutrients, stimulates the growth of healthy intestinal bacteria, and promotes their synthesis of B vitamins. It is a very effective antioxidant and free-radical deactivator, and reactivates vitamin E that has been oxidized during

"Humans taking large doses of vitamin C will not necessarily get a fall in serum cholesterol—indeed, they may get the reverse, because they are mobilizing their arterial cholesterol. The actual serum level is not relevant when they are taking the vitamin, since the cholesterol is being channeled in the right direction—away from the arteries."

Dr. Constance R. Spittle, British pathologist, letter to the editor of *Hospital Tribune* (1971)

peroxide deactivation. It also increases the production of lymphocytes, the defense cells of the immune system.[363]

Among vitamin C's special functions, it combats both organic and inorganic poisons. These include mercury, cadmium, lead, arsenic, chromium, and benzene; poison oak and poison ivy; snake, spider, and insect poisons; viral and bacterial toxins (including tetanus and botulism); and many industrial contaminants and pollutants.[370] It offers significant protection against radiation.[371] It can protect against, or overcome, numerous diseases and disorders, including arthritis, rheumatism, poliomyelitis, hepatitis, herpes, mononucleosis, rabies, smallpox, tuberculosis, whooping cough, pneumonia, leprosy, typhoid, typhus, dysentery, cancer, leukemia, atherosclerosis, many forms of heart disease, influenza, and, of course, the common cold.[365, 366, 367]

Why, one must ask, are these conditions not routinely treated with massive doses of ascorbic acid? The answer is simple: because we are still living in an era of ignorance and professional prejudice. It is well-accepted, even in orthodox medicine, that ascorbic acid simultaneously decreases the toxicity of most drugs and antibiotics and increases their effectiveness. Still, this vitamin is rarely if ever given with them. Its value for combatting infection is even denied. Many physicians and scientists have stated that giving patients several hundred milligrams of ascorbic acid has had little or no effect against the common cold or other diseases. Since all the successful work with this substance used dosages in the thousands and tens of thousands of milligrams, their results are not surprising. *

Dosage is important in both normal and abnormal situations. Ascorbic acid, being a water-soluble material, is not stored in the body. It saturates the tissues and passes out of the body in the urine, feces, and sweat. It needs to be replaced constantly. If a person is deficient in this vitamin, as most people are, his or her tissues will soak up about 4,000 mg before any is excreted.[67] Many opponents of megascorbic doses insist that after saturation is reached, nothing can be gained by taking more, because it will only be lost in the urine. The purpose of large doses, however, is not merely to saturate the tissues, but to flush them with the substance, so that it is constantly moving through them and out through the excretory organs. When ascorbic acid neutralizes toxins and renders them soluble, they must be washed out of the tissues and excreted. As ascorbic acid is used up, much of it is

"Vitamin E is the principal fat-soluble antioxidant, and vitamin C (ascorbic acid) is the principal water-soluble antioxidant. They probably cooperate in providing protection for our bodies and slowing the aging process."

Dr. Linus Pauling,
*Executive Health*, Volume 10

---

* It has frequently been cited that, in 1942, Cowan, Diehl, and Baker proved that "massive" doses of vitamin C had no effect on either the incidence or the severity of the common cold. The actual dosage used by these investigators was only 200 mg daily.[49]

metabolized into dehydroascorbic acid. If too much of this substance accumulates, it can have several undesirable side effects. When large doses of it are injected into rats, for instance, it can produce diabetes-like symptoms. [259, 362] Constant replacement of ascorbic acid keeps the metabolites and neutralized toxins flushing out of the body. The ascorbic acid acts like a detergent and rinsing aid. To say that extra dosages are wasted through excretion is like saying that soap and water are wasted because they only go down the drain. Furthermore, it is desirable to have ascorbic acid in the urine. Certain kinds of bladder cancer are caused by chemical reactions in the urine which form carcinogens, such as cinnabaric acid and N-nitroso compounds. Ascorbic acid in the urine prevents these reactions. [233]

Modern nutritionists are beginning to realize that the human body requires daily dosages of vitamin C ranging between 5,000 and 15,000 mg. There are several pertinent facts about megascorbic dosaging, however, that are usually overlooked.

Further back in our evolutionary history, ascorbic acid was produced in the liver or kidneys, and was transmitted directly to the bloodstream. The intestinal tract did not become the route of absorption until we had lost the ability to synthesize our own. Even then, it was mostly obtained from tropical fruits and raw, freshly killed meat. High-dosage tablets of vitamin C can be distressful to sensitive stomachs. When a tablet is swallowed, it dissolves slowly, often incompletely, concentrating its acidity in one portion of the stomach. If this happens, it will not be well-absorbed and may result in acid stomach and diarrhea.

A more comfortable alternative is powdered vitamin C. It can be used as a lemon or vinegar substitute, sprinkled on fish, salads, vegetables, etc. One level teaspoonful of ascorbic acid equals about 3,000 mg. Two teaspoonfuls of the powder, dissolved in a quart of drinking water, will make a refreshing, slightly tangy beverage. Each eight-ounce glass will provide 1,500 mg of the vitamin. The light acidity makes this drink more thirst-quenching than plain water, especially during hot weather. The exact dilution and acidity can be varied to suit the individual's taste. Your sense of taste is the best judge of how much acidity your stomach will tolerate. At first, an unsweetened, acidic drink may seem strange to some people, especially to those with a sweet tooth. But most people quickly acquire a taste for it; even a craving. Many people lose their addiction to sweets after using C-water for a week or so. If you don't like the tartness, add a little honey or fructose. Ascorbic acid should be taken throughout the day to maintain it at a fairly high level in the body tissues and to keep it flushing through the body. Most people find it difficult to remember to take some vitamin C every few hours. If it is already mixed in drinking water, you don't have to think about it. Since ascorbic acid increases the flow of urine, more water is needed with it anyway.

Ascorbic acid can also be added to fruit juice or wine, but should then be drunk soon after mixing, since juices and wines contain enzymes that rapidly decompose vitamin C. There is even some decomposition of the vitamin in plain water if it is allowed to sit too long, especially at room temperature or exposed to direct sunlight. Prepare only as much as you will use within about eight hours, and keep it refrigerated if possible. Because vitamin C has a low pH (is acidic) and is an antioxidant, it keeps fruit juices fresh longer. Don't add vitamin C to champagne or carbonated drinks. They will fizz and go flat. If you favor lemon with tea, add a pinch of vitamin C instead.

Natural vitamin C, derived from rose hips or acerola cherries, is available in most health-food stores at a rather high price. Synthetic vitamin C is much less expensive. Manufacturers of natural vitamin C would have us believe that their product is better than the synthetic. But it is not. The synthetic is produced from a natural substance (glucose) by essentially the same steps that take place in nature.[260]

Some vitamin C tablets contain added rutins and bioflavonoids. These substances are often found in nature with ascorbic acid, and are sometimes regarded as part of the vitamin-C complex. They strengthen cell membranes and capillaries, and in some ways potentiate the effectiveness of the vitamin. If the vitamin C that contains them is not too expensive, it is worth buying; but generally it is cheaper to buy them separately and take them with ascorbic acid. Some brands contain 500 mg of ascorbic acid and 100 mg of mixed bioflavonoids per tablet. If you are using these as the sole source of vitamin C in the dosages that we have suggested, you'll obviously get more than the recommended 100 mg of rutins and bioflavonoids. You can take 200 to 400 mg during illness, or prior to exposure to excessive pollution or radiation. Rutins and bioflavonoids are found in some fruits and vegetables. Citrus-fruit pulp and bell peppers are excellent sources.

Citrus fruits are also supposed to be good sources of vitamin C, but actually they do not come anywhere near to fulfilling our needs. An eight-ounce glass of fresh orange juice contains little more than 100 mg. Grapefruit has even less. A freshly picked, sun-ripened bell pepper may contain up to 300 mg. A large, fresh guava—common in Mexico, rare in the U.S.A.—may contain 1,000 mg.[67] When a fruit is picked, its vitamin C begins to oxidize. By the time commercial produce reaches us, most of its ascorbic acid has been depleted. Oxidation occurs even more rapidly when the fruit is juiced. Unless you have a back yard full of ascorbic-acid-rich fruit trees, you cannot obtain adequate amounts of vitamin C without resorting to supplements.

Many interactions occur between one nutritional component and another. When larger amounts of one are taken, certain others have to be increased. Vitamin C can wash harmful elements, like cadmium, lead, and aluminum, from the tissues, but it will also leach out essential trace minerals and water-soluble B vitamins. This presents no problem if all of these components are supplied abundantly every day (daily requirements of vitamins and minerals are discussed in Chapter 6). Recent reports indicate that vitamin C supplements taken with meals can interfere with the assimilation of vitamin $B_{12}$.[83] Except for the use of small amounts of vitamin C as a lemon or vinegar substitute on fish or vegetables, it is best to take ascorbic acid between meals, preferably as C-water.

Some people avoid the acidity of ascorbic acid by taking it as sodium ascorbate. This should not be done by anyone who has high blood pressure, or is on a low-sodium diet. Even for a normal person, this is too much sodium if the megascorbic doses suggested here are taken. If the diuretic properties of ascorbic acid taken before bedtime result in a full bladder that interrupts sleep, switch to sodium ascorbate for supplements two hours before bedtime. Sodium causes the tissues to retain water and inhibits the diuretic effects of ascorbic acid. Some bottles of tablets that are labeled vitamin C are actually sodium ascorbate. Always check the fine print on the side of the label to see if it is the sodium salt.

Vitamin C is also available as the ascorbate of essential minerals, including calcium, magnesium, zinc, manganese, and selenium. Like sodium ascorbate, these have no acidity. Minerals as ascorbates are very easily assimilated, and the vitamin is more stable in this form. When taking these ascorbates, you must pay attention to the proportions of minerals to ascorbate that are obtained. A mineral ascorbate molecule contains approximately one part of the mineral to nine parts ascorbic acid. A 500-mg tablet of calcium ascorbate, then, would contain 50 mg of calcium and 450 mg of vitamin C. To get 15,000 mg of vitamin C daily, you would have to take 16,500 mg of the ascorbate. This would supply about 1,650 mg of calcium, a good average supplemental intake. However, this much of some of the other minerals may be far more than is desired, or even safe. (Ideal mineral dosages are discussed in Chapter 6.)

Several concerns about massive vitamin-C dosages have been expressed by a few scientists and physicians.[147] Not all of these are without validity, but they should present no serious problems if one is aware of them. High levels of ascorbic acid excreted in the urine may give false readings in some tests for glycosuria. If you are to undergo such tests, advise your physician of your use of the vitamin. Then dosages can be temporarily reduced, or a different testing method can be used. Large dosages of vitamin C can also interfere with anticoagulant therapy that uses heparin or coumadin drugs. This also should be discussed with the physician.

Large amounts of ascorbic acid can increase iron absorption more than may be desired in nonanemic or nonpregnant persons.

This effect can even be dangerous if iron supplements are taken (see Chapter 6). Although vitamin C facilitates the assimilation of iron and calcium, it may inhibit the absorption of some trace minerals, at least in chickens.[147] For this reason also, the vitamin should be taken between, rather than with, meals.

Because some ascorbic acid is converted to oxalic acid, it has been feared that a high intake of the vitamin and of calcium may lead to calcium oxalate urinary stones. Although there have been no actual reports of this, adequate intake of magnesium and vitamin B6 should eliminate the possibility.[77, 115] Many studies have shown that high ascorbate intake actually lessens the incidence of oxalate stones and other types of urinary gravel.[369]

Several animal studies and one clinical study have indicated that massive vitamin-C dosages may interrupt pregnancy or have an adverse effect on the fetus. These studies are limited, inconclusive, and contradicted by other studies. There is, in fact, much more evidence that megascorbic dosages are beneficial to both mother and fetus.[373] Because of the unfavorable reports, however, we recommend that pregnant women take the question up with their doctors.

It is possible that long-term use of high dosages of vitamin C or any nutrient may result in a conditioned deficiency, that is, a relative lack of responsiveness to normal dosages. Although this problem is likely to happen only in old or ailing persons whose abilities to assimilate and make use of nutrients is diminished, a person who has been taking large supplemental dosages of certain nutrients for a long time should probably not stop suddenly—if stopping is at all necessary—but should taper off gradually over a period of weeks or even months. It is generally the practice in the Soviet Union to prescribe supplements for three to four weeks, then to switch off for the same amount of time. This assures that the patient will retain the ability to derive maximum percentages of components from normally nutritious diets.

*Tocopherols (Vitamin E).* Vitamin E is one of the most misunderstood nutritional materials, largely because it has been falsely promoted as the "sex potency" vitamin. It is actually much more generally valuable than that. Let's take a look at some of the misconceptions and myths, and see what this vitamin does and doesn't do.

Vitamin E refers to any of the several isomeric forms of compounds of the tocopherol group, including alpha, beta, gamma, delta, epsilon, zeta, and eta-tocopherols. These are oil-soluble substances found in egg yolks, wheat germ (and other grains), unrefined vegetable oils, nuts, seeds, leafy vegetables, and milk. Alpha-tocopherol is the most biologically active isomer of the series, but the others may be necessary for the proper functioning of this vitamin. It has been reported that the delta and gamma isomers are more potent antioxidants (at least in the test

> "It is my opinion that the authorities are wrong about vitamin E as they were about vitamin C."
>
> Dr. Linus Pauling,
> *Executive Health*, Volume 10

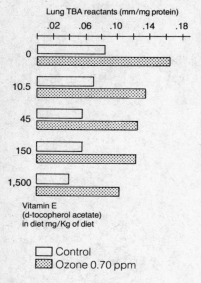

Lung TBA reactants (mm/mg protein)

.02  .06  .10  .14  .18

0

10.5

45

150

1,500

Vitamin E
(d-tocopherol acetate)
in diet mg/Kg of diet

☐ Control
▨ Ozone 0.70 ppm

*Vitamin E and lung-damage protection.*

Smog contains several chemicals which cause peroxidation of lipids and result in damage to cell membranes. Since smog is now a fact of life for many and probably shortens lifespans, an important question is whether antioxidants in the diet can offer any protection. There is some indication that they can.

Fletcher and Tappel studied the protective effects of antioxidants in the diet in rats which were exposed to high levels of oxidants. The results shown here are for rats fed vitamin E ($\alpha$-tocopherol) and exposed for five days to 0.70 ppm ozone (maximum oxidant levels during smog alerts in Los Angeles are about 0.80 ppm ozone). "Lung TBA reactants" represents malonaldehyde (*n* moles/mg protein) and reflects the amount of lipid-peroxidation damage in the lungs.

tube) than the alpha form. The entire series can be found where the vitamin occurs in nature, and in supplements labeled "mixed tocopherols."

In 1922, Evans and Bishop demonstrated that a deficiency of vitamin E produced sterility in rats. Consequently, the substance was promoted as "the sex vitamin." For the most part, it has been greatly overrated as such, but it does have several beneficial influences on sexual health. The greatest concentration of the vitamin is in the anterior pituitary gland, where it influences the production of male sex hormones. It also protects these hormones and other vital substances in the body against oxidation. It decreases the oxygen requirement of the cells and improves the cardiovascular system. It is necessary for the synthesis of coenzyme Q, which is essential in the respiratory sequence by which most energy is produced. By inhibiting the peroxidation of unsaturated fatty acids in the body and by minimizing oxygen starvation in the tissues, vitamin E may also help prevent the accumulation of arterial cholesterol. Cholesterol tends to collect in areas where oxygen supply is poor, and intact polyunsaturates assist in dissolving them. For all the above reasons, vitamin E may help improve a person's sexual capacity, but only if it has been low because of a deficiency. Extreme deficiency can lead to weakened muscle tissues, disorders of the reproductive system, irreversible degeneration of the testes, sterility, miscarriage, stillbirth, and heart disorders. The vitamin has been used to relieve menopause difficulties, including backache, excessive menstruation, hot flashes, high blood pressure, and muscular discomfort.

Vitamin E has several properties that indicate that it may be valuable as an antiaging drug. It is a very effective antioxidant and free-radical deactivator. At present, it is the only known antioxidant that can prevent lipid peroxidation within the microsomes and mitochondria. It further lowers lipid peroxidation by aiding in the efficient use of oxygen. It protects cell membranes, and helps prevent some types of anemia and cancer. The beneficial influences that it has on the heart, the hormonal system, and cholesterol levels can do much to prevent premature aging and untimely demise. There is very little evidence that vitamin E by itself can extend human lifespan beyond the average maximum, but it may be able to do so when used in combination with other antioxidants. Although much more study is needed, here are some of the findings which point in that direction.

*In vitro* embryonic fibroblast cultures normally reproduce for about fifty generations (the Hayflick Limit) and then die. When Lester Packer added vitamin E to the culture medium, the cells reproduced for as many as 120 generations,[252] perhaps because the vitamin reduces the oxidation caused by the high percentage of oxygen in the medium. Most cell-culture media contain about 20 per cent oxygen. Recently, Packer and Fuehr found that they could increase the number of generations by 25 per cent if the oxygen concentration was cut in half.[253]

Rats deficient in vitamin E die much younger than those receiving normal amounts of the vitamin, but large dosages do not significantly increase their maximum lifespans.

A 0.25 per cent concentration of alpha-tocopherol acetate in the nutritional medium of fruit flies increased their average lifespan by 12 per cent. In terms of human nutrition, this would equal about 1,135 milligrams per pound of food.[232]

In some Russian experiments, large dosages of vitamins A and E given to aging persons were reported to increase strength, cause a disappearance of facial wrinkles and headaches, improve sleep, and return color to gray hair.[294]

Vitamin E may prevent early death by preventing lipid peroxidation and free-radical formation in the body, and by combatting many forms of environmental pollution. It is strongly synergistic with other antioxidants, such as cysteine and selenium. Most of the vitamin E in our bodies is kept busy inhibiting the peroxidation of fats and hormones. Gerontologists believe that when other antioxidants and antiaging factors are simultaneously employed, the body's reserves of vitamin E may be free to play a part in slowing down the aging process.

The RDA of vitamin E is 20 to 30 IU (International Units; for vitamin E, an IU equals one milligram), which is about what a normal, wholesome diet provides if it includes plenty of fresh green, leafy vegetables and freshly milled whole grains. The vitamin is removed from white flour, and is destroyed by oxidation in all products as they rancidify during storage and shipping. As usual, our real requirements for this vitamin are far higher than the RDA. In supplying vitamin E, nature has again short-changed us, and the necessary channels of commerce have made matters worse. Even if we were to get our vitamin E from fresh wheat germ (about the best natural source), we would have to bloat ourselves with it to satisfy our actual needs. To obtain our full requirements of this vitamin, we must resort to supplements.

The question of ideal vitamin-E dosage is still open to debate. Much may depend on the individual diet. People who have a high fat intake should take more E than those who don't. Most nutritionists who are concerned with optimum health recommend at least 400 IU daily, and suggest that an extra 100 IU be taken for each tablespoonful of polyunsaturated vegetable fats consumed.[70] Many people who have been trying to preserve youth and promote longevity take 1,600 IU or more daily. Most of them have reported good results and no undesirable effects. Some scientists are now questioning the value and safety of such dosages. There is some doubt that the body can assimilate and utilize more than 400 IU per meal. Generally, vitamin E is regarded as nontoxic in dosages of 1,600 IU daily. There have been some recent media reports, however, of side effects, including chronic exhaustion and fatty liver, in some individuals after prolonged use of 1,600 to 2,000 IU daily. If unexplainable exhaustion occurs and continues, it is best to stop using supplemental vitamin E for several weeks, and resume supplementation with smaller doses after the symptoms have completely disappeared. It would also be wise to see a physician who is acquainted with these reports, and have him test for liver changes.

Extremely large dosages of vitamin E given to laboratory animals can produce toxic effects on the adrenal, thyroid, and sex glands. There is one recorded case of a person who took 4,000 IU of synthetic vitamin E for three months and suffered diarrhea and sore membranes.[70] We recommend that you not take more than 1,600 IU daily for more than a few weeks at a time. The ideal dosage appears to be somewhere between 800 and 1,200 IU. If other antioxidants—particularly ethoxyquin, BHA, or BHT— are being taken, it is better to lean toward the lower dosage.

The important thing is to get the most out of the vitamin E that we take. It is most effective when taken with other antioxidants, expecially selenium and cysteine. If you read the labels on several different brands of vitamin E, you will see that some contain *d*-tocopherol and others *d,l*-tocopherol. The *d* and *l* are initials for its two isometric forms, dextrorotary and levorotary. The *d,l-* product contains equal portions of *d-* and *l*-tocopherol. Many health enthusiasts are willing to pay the higher price for *d*-tocopherol, because they know that it is naturally derived, whereas the less expensive *d,l*-product is made synthetically. But they are not gaining any special benefit from the natural vitamin that cannot be had from the synthetic. Although only the *d*-form is biologically active, about forty-two per cent of the *l*-molecule is converted to the *d*-structure in the body. The measurement IU refers to the amount of biological activity, not the amount of the substance. One milligram of *d,l*-alpha-tocopherol equals one IU of vitamin E activity, whereas one milligram of *d*-alpha-tocopherol equals 1.36 IU. So, whether you take 100 IU of *d-* or *d,l*-tocopherol, you still get the same amount of usable vitamin E.[231]

Some longevists feel that it is wise to take both alpha and mixed tocopherols, perhaps altering from one meal to the next.

Since vitamin E is an oil-soluble material, it is stored in the tissues. If you don't take it for several days, or even weeks, it will not matter as it would with vitamin C and other water-soluble vitamins. Like all oil-soluble vitamins, E should be taken with meals that contain some fats or oils. These induce bile flow, which is necessary for assimilation. Vitamins A and D should be taken at the same time. Oil-soluble E is usually sold in sealed capsules. The vitamin is also available in a water-soluble form, as tablets, or as powdered vitamin-E acetate. Powdered E acetate has 50 per cent vitamin activity. 1,000 mg of it equals 500 IU.

Persons with high blood pressure, overactive thyroid, or heart damage from rheumatic fever should not take high dosages of vitamin E without the supervision of a physician. In these situations, they will usually be started on 30 IU for the first month, with a 30 IU increase every month, until the desired dosage is reached. Diabetics on insulin should also be under medical supervision when taking more than 30 IU of vitamin E supplements daily. [7, 82, 343]

*Sulfur Amino Acids and Other Sulfhydryl Compounds.* Nutrition books often neglect to mention sulfur. In its natural dietary form, sulfur is an essential mineral and a powerful aid in protecting against pollution and radiation. On top of that, it has now been found to extend lifespan.

Amino acids are the substances from which the body constructs its proteins. Most amino acids are constructed only of atoms of carbon, hydrogen, oxygen, and nitrogen; the few which also contain sulfur, such as cysteine, taurine, and methionine, function as antioxidants, free-radical deactivators, neutralizers of certain toxins, and aids to protein synthesis. In most of these capacities, cysteine is the most effective of these sulfur amino acids.

Although cysteine and others of this group are found in some foods, such as eggs, cabbage, muscle meats, onions, and garlic, many longevists supplement their diets with 500 to 2,000 mg of L-cysteine hydrochloride, which can be especially valuable in the polluted environments in which most of us live. Cysteine neutralizes acetaldehyde, a dangerous irritant and toxin occurring in cigarette smoke and smog. When rats were given doses of acetaldehyde large enough to kill 90 per cent of the untreated control group, those which had been treated with L-cysteine thirty minutes prior had an 80 per cent survival rate. [355]

Cysteine hydrochloride has a pleasant, salty, garlic-like taste, and can be sprinkled on food in place of salt. One level teaspoonful equals about 3,000 mg. It tends to absorb moisture from the atmosphere, and should be stored in a rust-proof container.

Methionine plays an important role in detoxification. It supplies the methyl group that converts a toxic substance, guanidine, to a relatively nontoxic chemical, methyl-guanidine. Chronic fatigue and exhaustion are sometimes caused by this toxin. When adequate methionine is supplied, improvement occurs almost immediately.

As well as being an antioxidant and free-radical deactivator, taurine facilitates the passage of potassium, sodium, calcium, and magnesium through the cell membranes. It also stabilizes membrane excitability, and may be important in the prevention of epilepsy. It is a very water-soluble substance, and therefore does not readily pass through the blood-brain barrier. However, it can be synthesized in the brain tissue from other amino acids. [278]

An average-size adult body contains about 140 grams of sulfur, of which about 850 mg is lost each day, and must be replaced. Eggs are about the richest food source of sulfur amino acids. They also contain the most perfect balance of dietary protein.

---

Many people have stopped eating eggs because of the cholesterol scare. *The belief that eggs contribute to the accumulation of arterial cholesterol is utter nonsense.* Although this belief has been thoroughly disproved and repeatedly denounced by scientists, it is still perpetuated in the minds of laymen and many physicians. Eggs do contain cholesterol, but they also contain lecithin, iron, sulfur, zinc, and various trace minerals which keep cholesterol from accumulating on the arterial walls, and provide the necessary materials to convert it into steroid hormones and other useful substances. [269, 376, 378]

---

> "The elimination of eggs and butter from the diet of a healthy person, merely because they contain cholesterol, is an extreme measure which can scarcely be justified on the basis of present knowledge."
>
> Dr. Edmund S. Nasset, University of Rochester physiology professor, *Chemical and Engineering News* (1972)

Generally, we derive our sulfur requirements from sulfur amino acids. The consensus of biochemical opinion is that humans cannot use elemental sulfur to make sulfur amino acids. However, Dr. Carl C. Pfeiffer, Director of the Brain Bio Center at Princeton, claims that we can also use elemental sulfur, because intestinal bacteria convert it to hydrogen sulfide. Perhaps this conversion explains the efficacy of the old-time sulfur and molasses tonic. Pfeiffer recommends that a No. 1 gelatin capsule be filled with flowers of sulfur (sold at drug stores) to provide 200 mg of the element. Since it is not entirely certain how effective this approach is, we suggest that the mineral be mainly supplied through dietary and supplemental sulfur amino acids. One egg contains about 65 mg of sulfur. One gram (1,000 mg) of cysteine hydrochloride (monohydrate) contains approximately 180 mg of sulfur. [278]

It has been found that some vitamin C in the body is converted to ascorbic acid-3-sulfate. [147] This suggests that large dosages of vitamin C may place demands on our sulfur reserves. Legumes, such as soybeans, are poor in sulfur amino acids. *Vegetarians who do not eat a lot of eggs should take extra sulfur.*

For many years, sulfur amino acids and related compounds have been used to protect against radioactivity. Radiation does much of its damage by removing electrons from water molecules and thus forming hydroxyl radicals, which unite to produce peroxides. These inactivate catalase and other enzymes by damaging sulfhydryl (-SH) groups in them. Sulfur amino acids and other sulfhydryl drugs provide sulfhydryl groups as sacrificial material to combine with peroxides and free radicals, so that the sulfhydryl groups of the enzymes are protected. The amino acids are then converted into harmless, or even useful, substances. [56, 298]

> "We must educate people away from the dangerous idea that you can control heart disease by not eating foods such as eggs, butter, and milk. This oversimplified idea is totally wrong."
>
> Dr. Linus Pauling, *Vitamin C and the Common Cold*

Sulfur amino acids also chelate various metals in the tissues. Excesses of certain metallic cations, such as copper ($Cu^{2+}$ and $Cu^+$), in the tissues promote the longevity of free radicals and enhance the formation of cross-linkages. Sulfur amino acids chelate these metals, so that they are easily excreted. It is also believed that sulfur amino acids may bind and stabilize portions of the DNA that are not covered by histones. As a result, not only is gene damage reduced, but, if damage does occur, the process of replication may be arrested, so that the DNA helix can be repaired before the damage-induced alterations are replicated.

Another sulfhydryl compound that shows much promise as a life-extension drug is 2-mercaptoethylamine (2-MEA), also known as cysteamine. In 1957, Denham Harman of the University of Nebraska added 2-MEA to the diets of male AKR mice and female C3H mice. These strains of experimental mice have been

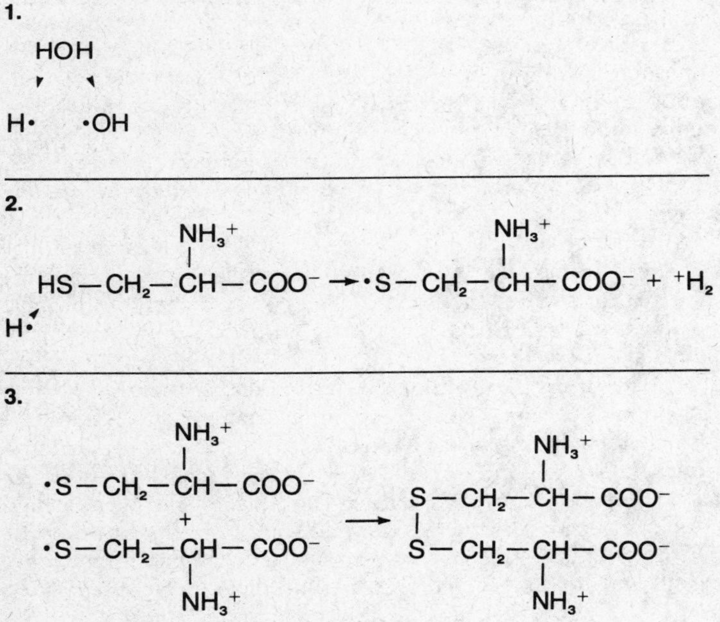

**1.**

HOH

H·   ·OH

---

**2.**

$$HS-CH_2-\overset{\overset{\displaystyle NH_3^+}{|}}{CH}-COO^- \longrightarrow \cdot S-CH_2-\overset{\overset{\displaystyle NH_3^+}{|}}{CH}-COO^- + {}^+H_2$$

H·

---

**3.**

$$\cdot S-CH_2-\overset{\overset{\displaystyle NH_3^+}{|}}{CH}-COO^-$$
$$+$$
$$\cdot S-CH_2-\underset{\underset{\displaystyle NH_3^+}{|}}{CH}-COO^-$$

$\longrightarrow$

$$S-CH_2-\overset{\overset{\displaystyle NH_3^+}{|}}{CH}-COO^-$$
$$|$$
$$S-CH_2-\underset{\underset{\displaystyle NH_3^+}{|}}{CH}-COO^-$$

*Cysteine as a terminator of free-radical reactions.*

Cysteine may be converted into cystine during the inactivation of free radicals by the following process. (1) Radiation can cause free-radical formation when it is absorbed by a chemical bond, in this case, water. The extra energy splits the molecule into two free radicals. (2) Cysteine is struck by a free radical of hydrogen. Ordinary molecular hydrogen is formed, leaving behind a cysteine free radical. (3) Two such cysteine free radicals may then combine to form a disulfide bridge and produce cystine, a useful compound.

developed to die prematurely; the AKR of lymphatic leukemia, the C3H of mammary cancer. Harman achieved a 20 per cent lifespan increase over the controls (7.5 to 9 months) with the male AKRs, but no increase with the C3H females.[131] In another study, made in 1961, however, Harman increased the lifespan average of the C3H females by 26 per cent (14.5 to 18.3 months) using the same drug.[132] He achieved similar increases when he substituted a related drug, 2,2'-diaminodiethyldisulfide (cystamine). Takashi Makinodan of the National Institute of Health found that 2-MEA rejuvenates the immune system.[394]

Most of these sulfhydryl drugs also appear to restore protein synthesis to levels typical of young animals. This aspect of rejuvenation is discussed in Chapter 5. One sulfhydryl drug, 4-thiazolidinecarboxylic acid, when combined with folic acid, has been reported to increase lifespan. The combination also restores cell enzyme levels nearly to those found in young animals. Researchers Oeriu and Dimitriu found that protein in aged rats contains fewer free amino and carboxylic groups than in young animals. After treating aged rats (18 to 24 months old) for 21 days with this combination drug (also called folcysteine), the number of free amino and carboxylic groups in their protein was significantly higher than that of the controls.[246] Oeriu and his coworkers found that 250 mg of folcysteine, given intramuscularly three times a week, restores many enzyme systems in senescent human patients.[247]

In the Soviet Union, 200 mg of 2-MEA has been given for radiation sickness.[231, 394] This amount is suggested as a safe, yet effective, dosage for life-extension purposes. It should probably not be exceeded, especially if other sulfhydryl-group drugs are being taken as well.

Aside from their value as antiaging drugs, these sulfhydryl compounds also protect against various natural and unnatural forms of environmental pollution. As we have already mentioned, cysteine minimizes the effects of acetaldehyde. The chelating properties of sulfhydryl drugs can help remove heavy metal contaminants, such as cadmium and lead, from the tissues. We can notice that 2-mercaptoethylamine has a propensity for capturing and binding mercury. A portion of its name, *mercapto*, comes from the Medieval Latin *mercurium captans*, which means "capturing mercury." The radioprotective nature of the sulfhydryl compounds can lessen the effects of both man-made and cosmic radiation, which accelerate the rate of aging.[32, 109]

*Selenium.*　　Once thought to be a poisonous contaminant in food, selenium is now known to slow down aging and prevent heart disease, and it may help prevent cancer. Because this mineral is toxic in dosages that are only a few times larger than those required for optimum health, it has been warily ignored by most popular nutritionists. More information is now coming to light, however, and it is gradually being recognized as an essential trace element and one of the most significant factors in the control of the aging process.

Selenium is a powerful antioxidant and free-radical deactivator. It is a cofactor in the protective enzyme gluthionine peroxidase, which catalyzes the conversion of lipid peroxides to harmless hydroxy acids.[320] It detoxifies mercury, and prevents many substances from being converted into carcinogens. When taken with vitamin E, selenium enhances the efficiency of the vitamin by modifying its distribution in the tissues.[272] At the same time, vitamin E increases the body's tolerance to the mineral. Furthermore, the combination of the two improves the responses of the immune system by stimulating the production of antibodies.[17]

Because of both geological conditions and dietary habits, the intake of this mineral varies in different parts of the world. In the United States, where the average daily intake is 68 micrograms (mcg), the incidence of female breast cancer is 22.2 per 100,000. In the Philippines the average daily intake is 189 mcg, and the breast cancer rate is 5.4 per 100,000; in Japan it is 287 mcg and 4.0 per 100,000. Differences in the consumption of seafood, an excellent source of the mineral, are largely responsible for the differences in selenium intake between these nations.[29] High selenium intake has also been linked with low incidence of leukemia and of cancers of the stomach, colon, rectum, prostate, liver, and lungs.[334, 335, 337–339]

Because the amounts of selenium in soil and water vary so widely in the United States, it is difficult to calculate a typical average intake. In 1973, Raymond J. Shamberger and other researchers at the Cleveland Clinic Foundation made a comparative study of the relationship between amounts of selenium in soil and water and the incidence of cancer in 34 American cities. Those with more selenium had less cancer. They were Los Angeles, San Diego, Dallas, Fort Worth, San Antonio, Houston, Oklahoma City, Tulsa, Denver, Phoenix, Salt Lake City, Omaha, Wichita, New Orleans, Atlanta, and Birmingham. Those with less selenium and more cancer were Chicago, Cincinnati, Toledo, Dayton, Fall River, Brockton, Worcester, Youngstown, Albany, Rochester, Utica, New York City, Bridgeport, Providence, Allentown, Gary, and Wilmington.

In 1975, the Cleveland Clinic Foundation researchers found that heart disease, high blood pressure, and hardening of the arteries also were less prevalent in high-selenium areas.[340] The states in this study with the highest amounts of selenium in their soil and water were North Dakota, South Dakota, Wyoming, Nebraska, Colorado, and Kansas. Some soils in the West are so rich in selenium, which is concentrated by certain plants, that foraging animals ingest toxic levels of it and develop an often fatal disease called "blind staggers" or "alkali disease." There are mixed

"An increasing body of experimental and epidemiological evidence indicates that selenium possesses anticarcinogenic properties in animals and man."

Gerhard N. Schrauzer

reports from the best authorities about whether humans have received toxic doses from eating foods grown on selenium-rich soil. This seems to be more of a problem for animals than for humans, since we don't consume as much vegetation as cattle do, and the grasses they eat take up more selenium than most of our vegetables.[387] Also, cattle and sheep frequently munch on plants such as locoweed (*Astragalus* and *Oxytropis* species), which take up unusually large concentrations of the mineral.

When selenium is derived from food, it is usually in a chelated form, bound to an amino-acid molecule. In experiments with cancer prevention and life extension, several forms of selenium, such as sodium selenite and selenourea, have been used with good results. Selenoamino acids have also proven valuable.

1 Netherlands
2 U.K.
3 Denmark
4 Canada
5 Ireland
6 Switzerland
7 U.S.A.
8 Israel
9 Belgium
10 Australia
11 Sweden
12 Germany
13 Norway
14 Austria
15 France
16 Italy
17 Czechoslovakia
18 Hungary
19 Finland
20 Portugal
21 Poland
22 Hong Kong
23 Bulgaria
24 Greece
25 Yugoslavia
26 Taiwan
27 Japan

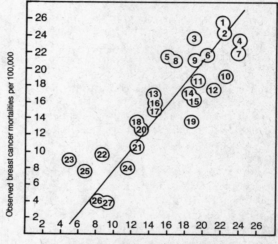

*Selenium intake and cancer prevention.*

Several studies have found low cancer rates to be correlated with high selenium. Correlations have been found with selenium levels in soil, selenium levels in the diet, and selenium levels in the blood. There are also studies on lab animals which indicate that certain tumors can be prevented by high selenium in the diet.

The correlation has been found for many types of cancer. The results shown here connect estimated selenium and zinc intake with the breast-cancer mortality rate in 27 countries. High selenium seems to be associated with lower cancer mortalities, but higher zinc levels tend to weaken the effect. A mathematical expression using both selenium and zinc was used to produce this graph. The probability that this kind of result (the straight line) happened by pure chance is less than one in ten thousand.

These studies suggest that if the average selenium intake in the U.S. were doubled, the breast-cancer mortality could be reduced to one-tenth the present level.

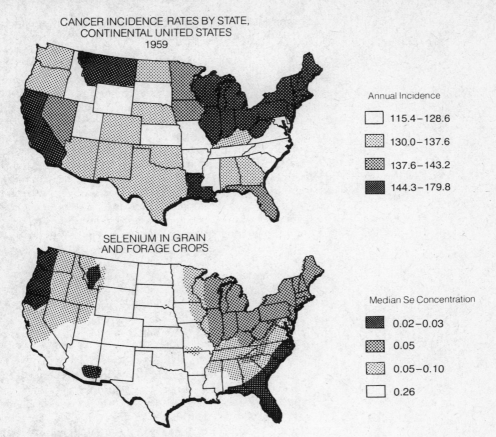

CANCER INCIDENCE RATES BY STATE,
CONTINENTAL UNITED STATES
1959

Annual Incidence

115.4–128.6

130.0–137.6

137.6–143.2

144.3–179.8

SELENIUM IN GRAIN
AND FORAGE CROPS

Median Se Concentration

0.02–0.03

0.05

0.05–0.10

0.26

*Selenium in crops and cancer prevention.*

One way to estimate the regional availability of selenium is to measure the amounts of it in forage crops. Such a measurement has been made for the continental United States (1959); the top map shows median selenium concentration (ppm) in grains and forage crops. If these selenium concentrations are compared with the bottom map, which shows annual cancer incidence per 100,000 persons, a significant inverse correlation is found: the cancer rate is lower where selenium levels are higher.

Those most frequently used are selenocystine, selenocysteine, and selenomethionine. These are virtually the same as cystine, cysteine, and methionine, except that the normal sulfur atoms of these amino acids are replaced by selenium atoms.

Raymond Shamberger reduced the incidence of induced cancer in mice by 15 per cent when he added 0.1 part per million of sodium selenite to their food. This represents 100 mcg per kilogram (kg) of food. When he raised this to 1.0 part per million (1 mg per kg), the incidence of cancer was lowered by 50 per cent.[256] Gerhard N. Schrauzer at the University of California in

COO⁻
|
+H₃N — CH
|
CH₂
|
CH₂
|
S
|
CH₃

*Methionine*

COO⁻
|
+H₃N — CH
|
CH₂
|
CH₂
|
Se
|
CH₃

*Selenomethionine*

San Diego reduced the incidence of induced mammary cancer in an inbred strain of susceptible mice (C3H females) from 82 per cent to 10 per cent by adding 2 parts per million of this compound to their drinking water (2 mg per liter). [166, 327, 328]

Discovering the maximum effective dosage of selenium that is not also dangerous has been a great concern of many longevists. Because of this uncertainty, even the most avant-garde nutritionists have been extraordinarily conservative in their dosage recommendations. Most have suggested a daily intake of 50 to 100 mcg, not to exceed 150 mcg. But since the average daily intake in Japan is 287 mcg, their caution has obviously led them into error. The LD50 (amount needed to kill 50 per cent of the test animals) for rats is 3 mg per kg of body weight if given all at once intravenously. [231] This would equal 210 mg for a 150-pound human, 1,400 times the overcautious 150-microgram limit. The cancer-prevention experiments described above employed dosages of 1 mg (1,000 mcg) per kg of food, or 2 mg per liter of water. A kilogram of food and a liter of water are about what a person might consume in a day.

Selenium is usually regarded as a toxic contaminant only when it exceeds 5 parts per million, or more than 5 mg per kg of food. [178] In a status report on selenium published in November 1976, the Food and Nutrition Board of the National Research Council stated,

"Available evidence suggests that a well-balanced diet furnishes about 60 to 120 mcg of selenium daily. Estimates of typical selenium intakes in the United States average about 150 mcg per day, and diet composites analyzed in Canada provide 98 to 220 mcg per day.... Should selenium supplements eventually be considered desirable for those persons living in low-selenium areas, or for those consuming vegetarian diets, a daily supplement of 50 to 100 mcg could probably be taken safely."

When considering this statement, one might bear in mind that the Board has rather consistently established RDAs (Recommended Daily Allowances) for vitamins and minerals far below the amounts required for ideal health, for example, vitamin C at 60 mg and vitamin E at 30 IU. Elsewhere in the report, the Board says, "Chronic selenium toxicity would be expected in human beings after long-term consumption of 2,400 to 3,000 mcg daily."

Many longevists take a minimum of 500 to 1,000 mcg of selenium supplements daily, and regard it as a safe but effective dosage. Some believe that the amounts needed for maximum protection against free radicals and lipid peroxidation are more likely to be in the range of 2,000 to 3,000 mcg daily. When taken with megadosages of ascorbic acid and vitamin E, the effectiveness of selenium is greatly enhanced, and tolerance to it is increased.[258] Also, if a person gradually increases his or her selenium intake, as we recommend for all nutritional supplements, greater tolerance to the mineral can develop. Since some signs of toxicity have been reported when selenium intake exceeded 5,000 mcg per kg of food, the proportions should be kept well below this level. This should present no problem when the mineral is obtained from natural sources. The most concentrated food source, high-selenium yeast, contains 5,000 mcg per kg, and no one is likely to consume that much yeast daily to the exclusion of all other foods. The toxicity of selenium is largely due to the fact that it can replace the sulfur in enzymes and other protein structures. Adequate supplies of sulfur, on the other hand, help to offset selenium toxicity.

A study made in high-selenium areas of Oregon revealed a somewhat high incidence of dental caries in children up to the age of ten. It is believed that the mineral may interfere with the beneficial effects of fluoride. [126] More research into this is needed, but it may be both unnecessary and unwise to give large dosages of selenium supplements to children.

Fruits and vegetables are usually poor sources of selenium. Whole grains, wheat germ, bran, onions, garlic, cabbage, broccoli, asparagus, mushrooms, tomatoes, corn, and soybeans may be good sources *if* they are grown on selenium-rich soil. Unfortunately, 70 per cent of the crops in this country do not contain adequate selenium. Eggs and other dairy products can also be good sources if the feed for the hens and cows is rich in the mineral. Tuna, sardines, herring, anchovy, and many other seafoods are likely to be more reliable sources, because the mineral distribution of the ocean is more homogeneous than that of the land, and because fish, unlike vegetables, are not necessarily restricted to the nutrients available in one location.

Brewer's yeast is generally regarded as the richest and most reliable food source of selenium, as any nutritional yeast would be if it were grown on a culture medium containing this element. Most yeast manufacturers do not indicate on the label what percentage of selenium, if any, is present, because very few people have cared about the mineral until recently, and most of those who had even heard of it regarded it as a contaminant. If selenium is not mentioned on the label, there may or may not be some in the product. We hope that the growing interest in selenium will prompt manufacturers to include selenium in the yeast culture and state the content on the label.

Selenates and selenites are usable forms of nutritional selenium. Although many longevists use sodium selenite drops, we hesitate to recommend them. Sodium selenite is an inexpensive and easily assimilated form of the mineral (90 per cent assimilation when dissolved in water), but overdosage can be dangerously toxic, and dosage is difficult to control.

*Deanol (DMAE).* During the past few years, deanol has attained some fame as a safe, natural stimulant. It also elevates mood, increases intelligence, and extends lifespan.

Most vitamins are present in foods in essentially the same structural forms in which they are used in the body. Some, however, occur in foods as other substances, from which the body manufactures the vitamin itself. These other substances are called vitamin precursors. The therapeutic administration of precursors, rather than the vitamins themselves, has in recent years begun to develop as a practical application of modern medicine.

Many dietary vitamins cannot permeate certain body sites, or are used up or otherwise destroyed before they can reach some parts of the body where they are needed. Some areas of the body have natural barriers that are designed to admit some substances while blocking the passage of others. Individual cells have protective membranes of this sort, and so do the tiny organelles within the cells. These membranes are two-way gates made up of complex phospholipid structures which allow most essential materials to enter in the correct proportions, prevent their loss from the cells, permit and assist the exit of waste products, and block the entrance of many unwanted substances.

Another membranous sentry system exists between the bloodstream and the brain. It is known as the blood-brain barrier (BBB). The brain is a very sensitive organ. Minute amounts of certain substances in the brain can cause radical changes in mood, personality, thought, and behavior. It is normal that there be water-soluble, toxic waste products in the circulatory system, for it is here that they are carried to the liver for detoxification or to the kidneys for excretion. But if they were to reach the brain, they could have disrupting effects. The BBB prevents such catastrophes.

Both the BBB and the membranes of the cells and organelles are marvelously designed systems, without which we could not live. In terms of the body's total needs, though, they do have their minor imperfections. Some substances that are needed within these highly guarded sites cannot gain entrance in any appreciable amounts. For this reason, precursors can be of great value. When a subject is given a precursor of lesser water-solubility than the desired compound, the precursor readily permeates the barrier, enters the site, and is converted by natural processes into the needed material. In a positive and beneficial sense, precursors may be regarded as biochemical Trojan horses.

The B-vitamin choline does not easily pass through the BBB. Aside from its role in maintaining the health and functions of the kidneys, liver, heart, lungs, and adrenals, choline is the material from which the body manufactures acetylcholine, which transmits electrical impulses in the brain and nervous system. Like its parent compound, choline, acetylcholine does not readily pass the BBB. No matter how much dietary or supplemental choline is received, or how much of the vitamin is present in the blood, a person can still have low amounts of acetylcholine in the brain. When there is a deficiency of this transmitter in the neurons of the brain, a person may display symptoms ranging from narcolepsy (brief attacks of sleep during waking hours), depression, sluggish behavior, slowed reflexes, and muddled thinking to nervousness, anxiety, and hyperkinetic patterns (usually in children).

Luckily, nature sometimes provides a precursor substance called dimethylaminoethanol (DMAE) that can pass the barrier to the brain, and be converted to choline and acetylcholine.[277] This vitamin precursor occurs naturally in fish, especially the more fishy-tasting varieties, such as sardines, herring, and anchovy. Hence it is appropriate that folk wisdom has always regarded fish as a brain food.

Aside from being a choline precursor, DMAE has several functions as an antiaging drug. It is a very efficient antioxidant and free-radical deactivator. It stabilizes lysosome membranes, preventing rupture of these scavenger bodies, which would result in leakage of collected toxins and protein-damaging enzymes. DMAE also appears to bring about repair of damaged cell membranes. How it accomplishes this is still not understood, although several explanations have been suggested. Paul Gordon of Northwestern University believes that the substance does not directly achieve the repair, but stimulates the cell's own repair capacities.[315] Since DMAE is the immediate precursor of choline, and since phosphatidal choline (also called lecithin; see p. 72) is one of the main phospholipids that make up cellular membranes, it is probable that the chemical does contribute directly to the structure of the membranes. Studies with radioactive tracers show that DMAE is rapidly incorporated into the cell membranes.[144] The compound also reverses the formation of the age-pigment lipofuscin in the membranes. Again, Gordon attributes this to a stimulation of the cell's regular scavenging mechanisms. Photomicrography reveals that DMAE speeds up the normal ejection of lipofuscin from the cells.[230]

DMAE also has several positive influences on red blood cells. Richard Hochschild, president of Microwave Instrument Company in Corona del Mar, California, and his coworkers have found that the addition of DMAE to whole blood stored for transfusion purposes doubles its storage life.[146] The substance also has an antisludging effect on circulating red corpuscles.[266] Sludging, the tendency of red blood cells to clump together like grape clusters, is a problem that happens with age. Sludging makes it difficult, or even impossible, for these oxygen-bearing corpuscles to pass through some of the smaller capillaries. If too much sludging occurs, some tissues may become oxygen-starved.

When Richard Hochschild added 86 mg of the acetamidobenzoate salt of DMAE to each liter of drinking water used by male A/J mice (a long-lived strain) that were already past their mean expected lifespan, the mean lifespan of the treated group was extended to 49.5 per cent over that of the controls, and the maximum lifespan to 36.3 per cent longer than that of the untreated animals.[144] Since a person will drink a liter or more of liquids daily, this experiment suggests that the human dosage needed for life extension is in the vicinity of 100 mg a day. The acetamidobenzoate salt of DMAE is produced by Riker Laboratories, Inc. under the brand name Deaner (the generic name is deanol), and is available by prescription. It is prescribed as a safe brain stimulant for hyperkinetic children, for others with learning and behavioral problems, and for narcolepsy. The usual therapeutic dosage is 300 mg daily, although deanol research pioneer Carl C. Pfeiffer recommends 400 mg.[266] Since it can cause insomnia, it is taken in the morning. Some people experience minor side effects, such as constipation, dull headaches, and tension in the neck, when they first start using deanol, but these usually disappear with continued use or reduction of dosage. When maximum results have been attained, the dosage is usually cut in half, otherwise the side effects may occur. There have been a few reports that deanol may cause heart irregularities in older persons already subject to them.[85] Otherwise, the drug is relatively safe and nontoxic. The dosage for life extension appears to be much lower than that used for brain stimulation. Lifelong daily use of such amounts should produce no disturbing side effect.

DMAE has other properties that are valuable for treating symptoms of aging. It improves mood levels of geriatric patients, relieves tension headaches and depression, serves as a safe CNS stimulant without having the undesirable side effects of the amphetamines, and apparently inhibits or even reverses signs of senile dementia. Unlike amphetamines, the drug improves appetite.

About 25 per cent of patients do not respond to deanol treatment, presumably because they do not have deficiencies of choline and acetylcholine. This is more likely to be the case if a person is a fish eater. People who obtain adequate choline and DMAE dietarily are less inclined to suffer from disorders that are treatable with deanol.[266] If they do display similar symptoms, some other problem is probably involved. Nevertheless, for life extension, even those who do not suffer from general choline or acetylcholine deficiencies should benefit from daily supplemental dosages of about 100 mg of DMAE in addition to adequate amounts of fish, especially sardines, herring, and anchovy. These are the same fish that Benjamin Frank recommends as rich sources of nucleic acids. Judging from Hochschild's mouse experiments, we can see that DMAE can have a significant effect on life extension even when use of it is begun fairly late in life.

Dimethylaminoethanol by itself is alkaline and somewhat caustic. Only salts and esters of it are used pharmaceutically. The acetamidobenzoate salt, produced by Riker for prescription sale, is an effective and well-utilized form. So is the bitartrate salt, which can be obtained from some chemical supply houses. The parachlorophenoxyacetic acid salt, also known as centrophe-noxine or meclofenoxate, is used in many European countries. Although it is essentially just another form of DMAE, it is often regarded, in life-extension literature, as a drug by itself, and since it seems especially effective in preventing and reversing the accu-mulation of the age pigment lipofuscin, we will consider it sepa-rately, in Chapter 3.

DMAE belongs to a chemical group known as alkylamino-alcohols. We mentioned earlier that some chemicals tend to propagate chain reactions of free-radical formation. Alkylamino-alcohols in general are free-radical chain propagators.[201] A person who is taking this substance should also take some of the other free-radical deactivators discussed in this book. These will promptly and harmlessly terminate the chain reactions. As we have already pointed out, combinations of various antioxidants and free-radical deactivators are usually more effective than any one drug alone.

## SYNTHETIC ANTIOXIDANTS
## AND FREE-RADICAL DEACTIVATORS
For some years now, people have been worrying about the chemical preservatives in commercial food. Now we are learning that some of these preserve not only our food, but our health and our youth as well.

All the substances we have discussed so far have been min-erals, amino acids, vitamins, and vitamin precursors found in nature, as well as a few closely allied derivatives of natural materi-als. We now turn to those substances that do not occur naturally, but must be synthesized by man. To many readers who are devoted to achieving health by means of "organic" nutrition, this may seem appalling. Modern man has mistreated his body so mercilessly with synthetic chemicals that most of us who have come to our senses about health have developed a zealous belief that only by adhering to nature's laws can we attain the state of glowing perfection that we envision as our birthright.

There can be no doubt, of course, that the way we have strayed from natural living has exacted a terrible price from us in terms of well-being. Our random dumping of synthetic drugs and chemicals into our systems has been careless, foolish, and often dangerous. We should certainly do our best to obtain all the materials necessary for life and health which are provided for us by nature. But at the same time we need not prejudice ourselves against the possibility that nature's creature of intellect, man, may successfully go beyond this scheme; that people may devise chem-icals which do not occur naturally in living organisms, but which can bring to our lives a state of health that nature alone could

"If it is natural to die,
then to hell with nature."
F. M. Esfandiary,
*Optimism One*

never offer. Nature, though amazingly efficient, is far from perfect; it has failed to provide some vitamin-like substances that our bodies require. Perhaps science must solve the riddles of nature's gaps, and fill in the blank spaces by inventing or discovering the missing molecules. Since we have already learned that nature has not provided enough of some vitamins to meet our real needs, we may reasonably suspect that some important substances have been left out of our foods entirely.

People have always accepted the aging process as natural and inevitable, mainly because they could find nothing in nature that could control it to any significant degree. Yet aren't the symptoms of aging similar to those of many nutritional deficiency diseases? It is conceivable that man may eventually devise a substance that can prevent or vastly slow down the aging process. When science creates such a drug, we will have to concede that it is a completely synthetic vitamin-like substance, unavailable from nature, but essential to life, and without which a person would suffer a cruelly disfiguring and debilitating death, prematurely, after less than a hundred years of life.

The potentials that several synthetic substances have for preventing certain degenerative diseases and increasing lifespan have often been discovered quite unexpectedly. Some of these chemicals had for many years been employed as commercial food preservatives, because they decrease the rate of oxidation in foods during storage. As a result of the widespread use of these preservatives, it was soon learned that they could also serve as antioxidants within the body. Gerontologists are now testing many of these chemicals on both animals and humans to learn how they can be most effectively used to retard aging. During the past few years, many people, on their own initiative, have been adding some of these chemicals to their armory of nutritional supplements. For the most part, beneficial results are being reported.

Although some of the synthetic antioxidants show much promise as life-extension drugs, we cannot recommend their use in the proportions employed in most animal experiments. Not enough is known about their far-reaching effects, although they appear to be safe and beneficial in moderate amounts. There have been a few reports of undesirable changes in the livers, kidneys, and thyroids of laboratory animals when given fairly large dosages of some of these drugs for a relatively long time. There have been similar reports about at least one natural antioxidant, vitamin E.

The side effects of most synthetics, like those of vitamin E, do not appear to result from any essential toxicity. Instead, they seem to occur because of either individual sensitivity or improper dosage. If the reader has decided to include any of these synthetics in his or her life-extension program, we suggest that the dosages be kept reasonably low and that function tests of the liver, thyroid, and kidneys be given periodically by a qualified physician, to detect any signs of unwanted changes. Even when one begins to use natural antioxidants and megavitamins, we urge that titration (gradual increments over a period of weeks or months, starting with very small dosages, until optimal dosage is reached) be practiced. The body must adapt to unfamiliar amounts of these nutrients and develop greater efficiency in assimilating, metabolizing, and making full use of them. This gradual approach is even more important when the system is being introduced to materials it has never before encountered.

In some respects, these substances may present a greater danger to laboratory animals than to humans. In one report, signs of kidney fibrosis occurred in rats that were given large dosages of one synthetic antioxidant. Large dosages of another crystallized in the animals' kidneys.[400] Unlike humans, rats excrete only small amounts of very concentrated urine in proportion to food intake.[129] A more diluted urine is not as likely to cause these problems. On the other hand, tests carried out during the relatively brief lifespan of a rodent cannot tell us what long-range effects these agents may have on human tissues.

We are not recommending the use of synthetic antioxidants, but we are trying to present the case for them fairly, and to give appropriate warnings about possible drawbacks. According to existing evidence and the consensus of opinion among longevists, a combination of small amounts of these synthetic agents and a full spectrum of natural ones is the safest and most effective approach.

*BHT and BHA.* Many crusaders for natural foods that are free of additives have expressed concern over the commercial use of BHT (butylated hydroxytoluene) and BHA (butylated hydroxyanisole) in many of our food products. However, experiments reveal that these chemicals, in the amounts used, have practically no systemic toxicity in either animals or humans. The LD50 (lethal dose for 50 per cent of the subjects) in rats is 1,600 to 3,200 mg of BHT, and 2,500 to 5,000 mg of BHA, per kg of body weight.[231] In a 150-pound human, the equivalent amounts would be between one-quarter and three-quarters of a pound. In a set of experiments conducted by Denham Harman at the University of Nebraska, mice that were fed normal diets containing five grams of BHT per kg of food (0.5 per cent) lived almost 50 per cent longer than the controls.[135] BHT and BHA are both antioxidants and free-radical deactivators. Harman conservatively states that BHT could add five years to the average human lifespan, but his own experiments suggest that it is more likely to add around thirty years.

Statistical drops in gastrointestinal cancers during the past few decades have been credited to the widespread use of these antioxidants as food additives. Lee W. Wattenberg of the University of Minnesota Medical School reduced the incidence of carcinogen-induced stomach cancer in mice from 100 per cent in

*BHT*

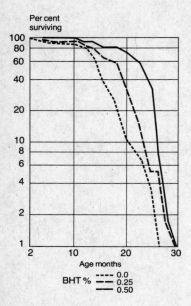

Per cent
surviving

Age months

BHT %  ---- 0.0
        -- - 0.25
        —— 0.50

*BHT and longevity.*
Harman found a number of anti-oxidants to be effective in increasing the mean lifespan of mice. The results shown here are for BHT.

the controls to 22 per cent by adding to the diet the same percentage of BHT that Harman used, and to 17 per cent by adding this much BHA.[396] The average American intake of BHT or BHA as food preservatives is between 1 mg and 2 mg daily. This amount gives some protection against stomach cancer, but our real needs for maximum anticancer and life-prolongation benefits are apparently much higher.

The anticancer properties of BHT are usually attributed to its inhibition of the formation of peroxides and cross-links in the cells and tissues. In recent years, two other anticancer characteristics have been ascribed to the chemical. During the early 1970s, two researchers demonstrated that the addition of 0.5 per cent BHT to the diet of albino hairless mice greatly reduced the incidence of skin cancer induced by ultraviolet light. At the end of 22 weeks, 30 per cent of the controls had developed squamous-cell carcinomas, compared to only 7 per cent of the animals receiving BHT.[24, 25]

BHT has also been found to be effective against lipid-containing viruses and bacterial viruses, both the DNA- and the RNA-containing kinds. Usually RNA viruses require different antibiotic agents than DNA viruses. *Herpes simplex* virus is one of the viruses whose infectivity is reduced by BHT. This virus not only causes genital infections, cold sores, and fever blisters in humans, but has also been linked with leukemia and several other kinds of cancer.[300] The chemical also gives protection against Newcastle disease virus, which attacks poultry.[33] It has been suggested that the antiviral activity of BHT is due to changes that it causes in the hydrophobic (repelling water and water-soluble substances) lipid membranes that coat these viruses.

Now that we know about BHT's antiviral properties, we can ask whether its function as an antioxidant and free-radical deactivator is the only way in which the drug can act against aging. Later we consider the so-called "slow virus" hypothesis of aging. If slow-acting, inapparent, but persistent viruses are responsible for increased autoimmune reactions and other, related degenerative aging changes, BHT may combat the viruses sufficiently to retard these changes.

There is much uncertainty among gerontologists and self-experimenting longevists about what the ideal human BHT dosage should be. In the successful anti-herpes experiments, dosages ranging from 20 to 100 mg per kg of food were used. Between 50 and 200 mg per kg is generally considered a harmless range. In his mouse life-extension experiments, Harman used 5,000 mg per kg, which may be more than is necessary or safe for humans, especially when other antioxidants are also being taken.

Concentrations of between 2,000 and 20,000 mg per kg of food can produce various changes in metabolism and cell functioning. It has not yet been discovered whether these changes are actually harmful. Some may even be directly related to the beneficial effects of the drug. For instance, workers at the Department of Poultry Science of the University of British Columbia in Vancouver found that when chickens were fed concentrations of 5,000 mg per kg of food, the number of circulating reticulocytes (immature red blood cells) in their bloodstreams was increased because the drug delayed the maturing of the young cells. [222] The Vancouver team suspects that the maturation of reticulocytes into functioning red corpuscles is related to the gradual loss of lipids from the cell membranes by normal but inevitable oxidation. BHT apparently inhibits the oxidation and loss of membranal lipids. Two other antioxidants, vitamin E and ethoxyquin, produced an even greater reticulocyte increase. None of these substances caused any other changes in blood composition, and no harm seemed to result from the reticulocyte increase. This much lipid-membrane protection could also be of considerable benefit in other kinds of cells.

In 1972, scientists at Loyola University reported that pregnant mice receiving 5,000 mg of BHT or BHA per kg of food often produce offspring with abnormal brain chemistry and behavioral patterns. [97] The committee that advises the FDA on food additives has expressed concern over the possibly harmful relationship between BHT and steroid hormones or oral contraceptives. They have asked for further studies of these combinations. Until more is known, pregnant women and persons on steroids or birth-control pills either should not take supplemental BHT or BHA, or should keep the dosage low.

Many self-experimenting longevists have been taking daily dosages of BHT or BHA ranging between 500 and 2,000 mg. To our knowledge, none have suffered any apparent ill effects. Most report improvements in health, energy, and general well-being. Most of them, however, are also taking other life-extension drugs and nutritional supplements. There are a few reports of individuals taking as much as 7,000 mg of BHT each day without evident harm, but tests for changes in kidney, liver, or thyroid functions were not given. [31]

BHT and BHA are used as preservatives in various food products, including breakfast cereals, enriched rice, potato chips, ice cream, baked goods, gelatin desserts, lard, shortening, candy, and chewing gum. The FDA allows amounts of these preservatives not to exceed 0.02 per cent of the food's total oil or fat content, that is, 200 mg per kg of fat or oil. This amount, also expressed as 200 parts per million, is permitted in shortening and other complete fats, whereas only 50 parts per million is allowed in cereals and potato chips. They do allow up to 1,000 parts per million of BHA in dry yeast, [404] but the supposition is that only small portions of yeast are consumed by most people. Since foods that contain these antioxidants usually make up only a tiny fraction of most Americans' diets, 2 mg a day is about the most that is obtained.

BHT and BHA are soluble in fats and oils, but not in water. BHT dissolves better in fats and oils than BHA, but the latter is believed to be more rapidly metabolized and less likely to cause kidney problems. The lethal dose of BHA for rats, we have already mentioned, is 50 per cent higher than that of BHT. Most longevists feel that 200 mg of supplemental BHT or BHA (not counting the smaller amounts that occur as commercial additives) is a safe daily dosage that should offer significant life-extension benefits, especially when used in combination with other antioxidants and free-radical deactivators. Larger amounts of these two substances may be perfectly safe and may provide additional benefits for most individuals, but we must strongly emphasize the importance of periodic medical monitoring when much larger dosages are taken for any length of time.

The limited solubilities of BHT and BHA have presented some problems for self-experimenters who have been attempting to incorporate these materials into their diets. If taken in capsules, these chemicals are not likely to be well-dissolved and distributed in the food content of the stomach. They will then be poorly assimilated, and, because of uneven diffusion, may be irritating to the stomach. If they are simply sprinkled on food like water-soluble supplements, they are unlikely to dissolve fully. Furthermore, the peculiar texture of BHT causes an annoying squeaky sound in the teeth when it is chewed.

There is a practical way to prepare BHT or BHA that can also be used with other lipid-soluble antioxidants, such as ethoxyquin or ascorbyl palmitate. Lightly warm 16 ounces of safflower (or similar) oil in a saucepan. Add two level teaspoonfuls of BHT or BHA (2,500 mg per tsp), and stir until all the crystals have dissolved completely. Let the oil cool for a few minutes, then pour it back into the bottle, cap it, and keep it in the refrigerator. Each teaspoonful of the oil now contains about 80 mg of the antioxidant; each tablespoonful, about 200 mg. There are about 25 tablespoonfuls of oil in a 16-ounce bottle, or about 60 teaspoonfuls. This much provides a family of four with a week's supply of 200 mg a day. It is best to prepare no more than can be used in a week or two, so that the antioxidant and the oil do not become oxidized. The oil can be used in salads or added to various dishes, but use no more oil than would provide the amount you have set for the antioxidant in your diet, and don't use it for frying (see page 75).

BHT and BHA are known to be generally synergistic (mutually potentiating) with other antioxidants. However, the results of one experiment by Harman seemed to indicate negative synergism between vitamin E and BHT. Male LAF1 rats were given various antioxidants, singly and in combinations. The effectiveness of each drug or combination was measured by the percentage of rats surviving at the age of 20 months. Of the controls, 8.7 per cent survived. Of those receiving 0.5 per cent (of dry food weight) of BHT, 61.1 per cent survived. Of those receiving 0.5 per cent vitamin E, 13.2 per cent survived. Of those receiving a combination of 0.5 per cent each of BHT and vitamin E, 32.8 per cent survived. [134] This reduction, from 61.1 per cent to 32.8 per cent, has led some longevists to conclude that BHT and vitamin E interfere with each other's actions and should not be taken together. [84] Harman's experiment appears to contradict other experiments with larger animals, such as chickens, cattle, and pigs. In these cases, BHT reduced vitamin E requirements and prevented E-deficiency damage. Since BHT is a liver-enzyme inducer, and since rat-liver enzymes are highly responsive to certain chemicals, the BHT in Harman's experiments may have accelerated the metabolism of the vitamin. Harman's figures suggest, however, that it was the E that interfered with the BHT, rather than the BHT with the E. Also, when Harman's rats received 1.0 per cent 2-MEA, 8.8 per cent survived (an insignificant increase over the 8.7 per cent of the controls), but when this much 2-MEA was combined with 0.5 per cent vitamin E, only 6.3 per cent survived. This suggests that 2-MEA plus vitamin E actually shortens lifespan.

Our own interpretation of these data is that the concentrations of vitamin E or BHT alone (5,000 mg per kg of food) were already quite high and bordering on the excessive level. Some of the reported negative side effects from too much vitamin E are similar to those from excessive BHT (e.g., liver changes). It is possible that the combination simply added up to an overdosage that shortened the lives of the more sensitive rats. The same explanation would apply to the vitamin E plus 2-MEA combination. Conservative dosages for each of these substances are suggested, especially if combined antioxidants are being taken. Harman's results could also be due to experimental error or unknown causes. More research on antioxidant combinations and ideal dosages is definitely needed.

Although BHT and BHA are classified GRAS (generally regarded as safe) by the FDA and are essentially nontoxic, some rare cases of allergic sensitivity to them have resulted in a mild dermatitis. This condition is not as likely to occur if all nutritional factors, especially vitamins A and C, are adequately supplied. We reiterate the importance of gradual titration when introducing such physiologically unfamiliar materials as BHT or BHA to the system. If dermatitis symptoms appear, reduce the dosage or stop it entirely.

*Ethoxyquin.* This substance is a quinoline-derived synthetic antioxidant produced by Monsanto Laboratories under the brand name Santoquin. It is used commercially to prevent the oxidation of sliced fruit and animal feeds. In a series of experiments conducted between 1968 and 1971, Denham Harman added 5,000 parts per million of ethoxyquin to the diets of mice,

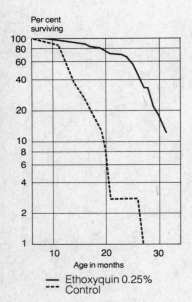

*Ethoxyquin*

*Ethoxyquin and longevity.*
Ethoxyquin fed to mice at 2,500 mg per kg of dried food (0.25 per cent) had a pronounced effect on the mortality rate. The diet contained 20 per cent casein (mild protein), and the amyloidosis usually resulting was practically eliminated by the ethoxyquin diet.

commencing shortly after weaning. In these experiments, the effects of other antioxidants, including BHT and 2-MEA, were also studied. These three compounds increased the mean lifespan of the animals by 30 to 45 per cent.

In one experiment, Harman compared the survival rate, after 20 months, of LAF₁ mice fed various antioxidants. The survival rate for the controls was 8.7 per cent. The survival rates for the treated animals were: BHT, 61.1 per cent; 2-MEA, 8.8 per cent; and ethoxyquin, 74.6 per cent.[135] In another experiment, conducted by Alex Comfort around 1970, C3H mice receiving similar amounts of ethoxyquin outlived the controls by about 18 per cent. The general condition and activity of the treated mice was better during aging than that of the controls. There was also a lower incidence of tumors than might be expected for this susceptible strain. The animals also grew to a lighter body weight than the controls and lost weight earlier in life.[44]

In a study by Dennis Eddy and Denham Harman, LAF₁ mice were maintained on a high casein diet to induce a high incidence of amyloid formation. Not only did the ones that received 2,500 mg of ethoxyquin per kg of dried food live longer, but the incidence of amyloidosis was reduced from 65 per cent to almost zero.[89] Amyloid is a starch-like protein that accumulates in the tissues of older animals and humans, and occasionally occurs as a complication of chronic infections and disorders, such as tuberculosis, leprosy, and rheumatoid arthritis. The fact that its structure is related to immunoglobin lends support to the theory that aging is due in part to a breakdown of the immune system. In 1964, it was found that senile plaques are composed of amyloid. These are microscopic formations which occur at the focal point of deterioration of the neural cells of the brain.[382] Amyloid is a by-product of senescence, but it may also be a cause of aging symptoms. It is certainly a measurable indication of aging progress.

The most surprising discovery about ethoxyquin is that it shows metabolic activity identical with that of vitamin E. In various experiments conducted at Monsanto Laboratories, ethoxyquin prevented symptoms of vitamin-E deficiency in animals, even when none of the vitamin was present in the diet, and when the type of diet would have required larger than usual amounts of the vitamin to avoid deficiency symptoms (for example, diets high in polyunsaturated fats).[235] This doesn't mean that you can stop taking vitamin E and replace it with ethoxyquin. All the biological functions of vitamin E are not yet known. Furthermore, there are possible dangers in prolonged use of large dosages of the drug. In the *Journal of Agriculture and Food Chemistry*, R. H. Wilson and F. de Eds reported the results of a study in which albino rats were given concentrations of 1,000 to 4,000 mg of ethoxyquin per kg of food. Although there were no outward symptoms or decreases in lifespan, autopsies revealed, in animals that had received concentrations of between 2,000 and 4,000 mg per kg, irregular areas of kidney fibrosis and signs of kidney disease, structural changes in liver cells, and possible thyroid damage.[400] Another report has linked large dosages of the drug with increased incidence of liver tumors in newborn mice.[361]

Ethoxyquin is approved by the FDA for human consumption, when used as an antioxidant for apples, pears, etc. In such uses, the concentrations would be quite low. The Monsanto Company manufactures the product only in Feed Grade (for animals) at present, but it meets all the FCC standards for Food Grade (for humans).

Individuals who have been using daily dosages of 1,000 to 3,000 mg report no apparent harm. None have taken the drug for more than two years, though, and their personal findings cannot indicate whether long-term use of these amounts is safe. If the self-experimenting reader intends to include this substance in his antioxidant program, it would be wise not to exceed 100 mg per meal, especially if a full range of other antioxidants is taken at the same time. Ethoxyquin is soluble in fats and oils, but not in water. It can be dissolved in warmed oil, like BHT.

## OTHER ANTIOXIDANTS
## AND FREE-RADICAL DEACTIVATORS

In addition to the substances already mentioned, several other antioxidants have shown experimental merit as antiaging drugs. Most of these have been used as food additives to prevent spoilage.

*Thiodipropionic Acid.*　　This white, crystalline powder, soluble in alcohol and in hot water, has been used as a stabilizer for vitamins and antibiotics, and to prevent flavor changes from oxidation in milk products and soybean oil. The FDA allows amounts that do not exceed 0.02 per cent of the fat or oil content of the food.[408] It is strongly synergistic with primary antioxidants, especially when citric acid is also present.[231] BHT, BHA, and many other substituted phenolic compounds function as primary antioxidants by terminating the propagation of chain reactions among free radicals that tend to accelerate oxidation. Thiodipropionates, such as thiodipropionic acid and dilauryl thiodipropionate, are secondary antioxidants. These break peroxides down to harmless substances before they can decompose to form additional free radicals.[79] Thiodipropionic acid has no known toxicity. Dilauryl thiodipropionate is regarded as generally safe by the FDA, but is on their list for further study.[405]

*Nordihydroguaiaretic Acid (NDGA).*　　This resinous substance, derived from a number of plants, including the creosote bush (*Larrea* and *Covillea* species) and the Guaiac gum trees (*Guaiacum officinale* and *G. sanctum*), was an antioxidant used in pie crusts, candy, lard, butter, ice cream, and canned whipped cream. Lard that contains 0.01 per cent NDGA can be stored at room temperature for up to 19 months without becoming rancid. [231, 407] NDGA has shown some effectiveness in extending the lifespan of Wistar rats. [35] In 1968, it was banned by the FDA because large dosages caused some kidney damage in rats. Some critics have argued that this problem may be peculiar to rats, since they excrete only small, concentrated amounts of urine. [129] Until further studies have been made, one would probably be wise not to use it as a dietary antioxidant. Some longevists have suggested the occasional use of creosote bush tea. This should be safe, if not effective, since NDGA is only slightly soluble in hot water.

*Ascorbyl Palmitate.*       This fat-soluble form of ascorbic acid has vitamin-C activity, is a powerful antioxidant, and is nontoxic. It is used in meat curing, and to prevent oxidative browning of cut apples and other fruit. [231, 403] Because of its solubility in fats and oils, it can be more effective in preventing lipid peroxidation than the water-soluble ascorbic acid. It is tasteless and can be sprinkled on foods, combined with blender drinks, or dissolved in salad oil. In addition to the usual megadosages of vitamin C, many longevists take 1,000 mg (1 teaspoonful) or more of ascorbyl palmitate each day.

*Other Antioxidants.*       Other antioxidants that have been tested, with varying degrees of success, in animal life-extension experiments include ammonium diethyl-dithiocarba-mate (DDC), propyl gallate, sodium hypophosphite, and sodium bisulfite. [134] Some of these have been employed in small amounts as food additives, and are regarded as safe in the minute percentages used. The FDA feels that further studies are needed before increased levels are used. This also applies to dosages that might be effective as antiaging drugs.

Several vitamins not yet mentioned have also been found to have some activity as antioxidants and free-radical deactivators. These are discussed in Chapter 6.

## The Use of Antioxidants

The wisest approach to using dietary supplements is to combine moderate amounts of various ones, rather than to use large quantities of any single agent. This approach would minimize the risk of toxic or allergic reactions to any one or more of the substances to which the individual may be sensitive, or which may be toxic in large amounts. It is best to use mainly those antioxidants that are vitamins, minerals, or similar substances that are already a part of our natural diet. If artificial chemicals, such as BHT, BHA, ethoxyquin, or the thiodipropionates, are also taken, dosages should be kept quite low, not exceeding a few hundred

"Antioxidant therapy alone should add five to ten years to the human lifespan; radiation protection alone should add two to five years; and success with protein missynthesis resorting should add five to ten years. The three protection mechanisms together will act synergistically, potentially producing a lifespan increase of thirty to forty years of youthful life."

Richard A. Passwater,
*Supernutrition*

milligrams of each. Fractional dosages should be used at first, to test for individual tolerance, and to allow the system to become accustomed to them. Gradual increments can be made over periods of weeks or months, until the optimal dosages are reached. Medical supervision, with periodic testing for changes in various body functions, is especially recommended for those who are experimenting with synthetic materials.

As we have seen, different antioxidants may have slightly different roles: as primary or secondary agents; as water-solubles or lipid-solubles; and as having activity in varied sites, e.g., microsomes, mitochondria, or cell membranes. For this reason, and because these substances are mutually potentiating, an appropriate mixture seems to be the most valuable. We cannot yet be certain what the ideal dosages and combinations are, but we have attempted, as far as possible, to examine existing data to get a fair indication of what amounts should be both safe and effective.

# Chapter Three

# Signs of Aging

## *Age Spots and Centrophenoxine*

*The dark brown spots that discolor the skin of aging people are a by-product of lipid peroxidation. These pigmentations also occur in other organs, including the brain, and may contribute to senescence. Fortunately, several drugs have been found that can literally wash these aging stains out of the tissues.*

Around 1958, several different laboratories independently discovered the presence of a yellowish-black, fluorescent, granular pigment in aging cells. This substance, known as lipofuscin, consists of 30 to 40 per cent lipids and large amounts of protein rich in valine and glycine. Analysis indicates that these materials are derived from the cell membranes in which they reside. They are usually more prominent in postmitotic cells; that is, cells which are fixed and do not normally replace themselves, such as those of the brain, neurons, muscle, and heart. Mitotic cells (those that do divide and replace themselves) may contain lipofuscin, but the accumulations are usually smaller because the pigment is diffused through each cell division.[14, 307, 374] Most evidence indicates that lipofuscin is a product of lipid peroxidation and free-radical reactions in the membranes of the cells and subcellular organelles. Malonaldehyde appears to be the agent that forms these age pigments.[42]

The major question about lipofuscin is whether the substance is a cause of aging or merely a symptom. Research, so far, has yielded much conflicting information. Lipofuscin accumulates in the cells and in some subcellular bodies, particularly the mitochondria and lysosomes.[315] Eventually, it can occupy up to 30 per cent of the cell's volume. It would seem that such large accumulations are likely to interfere with cell function.

Lipofuscin can occur in the cells of young persons, even newborn infants, but usually only in small, insignificant amounts. In a genetic disorder known as Batten's disease, however, such large deposits of the pigment build up in the brain cells of the child that the victim is blind by age five. There is then a continuous deterioration of brain function, followed by premature death.[307] Large amounts of the pigment also accumulate in the cells of progeria victims. Progeria is a tragic and mysterious disease in which the victim displays symptoms of aging very early in life and usually dies of apparent old age or age-related complications during his or her teens. The disease appears to be rooted in faulty DNA-repair mechanisms,[60] and there is no cure for it at this time. Strangely, while other aging characteristics progress, the progeric shows no signs of senile dementia. Lipofuscin seems to be a side effect, having no causal relationship to the disease or the progression of aging symptoms. In normal aging, however, buildups of the pigment in brain cells apparently contribute to a decrease in mental and motor abilities.

If large deposits of lipofuscin can strangle cells and obstruct their functions, they no doubt present similar problems in the mitochondria and lysosomes. Since all the cell's energy transformations take place in the mitochondria, it is likely that age pigment pileups here contribute to the losses of energy, muscular vitality, and reflex speed that befall the aged.

Since lysosomes are the scavengers of the cells, it is probable that lipofuscin in these organelles was picked up as garbage. It is not expected that it does any direct harm to these bodies, or that it causes rupture and leakage in their membranes. There is even some indication that it may strengthen the lysosome walls.[311] But it may also clog the membranal passageways through which wastes are collected. Certainly, it takes up space in these scavenger sacks that is needed for other, more toxic, garbage.

Although large accumulations of lipofuscin clog the cells and hamper their normal workings, there is some evidence that the substance, in lesser amounts, serves some protective purpose in the cell. Harold Brody of SUNY in Buffalo found that brain cells that lack lipofuscin deposits have a higher mortality rate than those which contain the pigment.[311] Perhaps lipofuscin is one of the body's tools for survival, but one that occasionally gets out of hand, especially during old age, when so many things go wrong and the body begins to turn against itself.

In the mid 1960s, K. J. Nandy and G. H. Bourne of Emory University in Atlanta observed that lipofuscin pigments become prominent in guinea pigs after four years of age. They treated a group of four- to six-year-old guinea pigs with daily dosages of centrophenoxine (80 mg per kg of body weight) for four to eight weeks, and found a notable decrease of lipofuscin in the brains of the animals.[238]

Centrophenoxine, also known as meclofenoxate, is a water-soluble powder derived from dimethylaminoethanol (DMAE) and para-chlorophenoxyacetic acid. It is nontoxic to humans and

*Centrophenoxine*

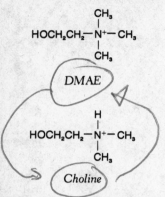

DMAE, the active part of deanol, is very close in structure to choline.

animals in the recommended dosages, and has been used clinically in Europe to treat reading problems, speech and motor dysfunction, psychosomatic asthenia of presenescence, failing memory, loss of concentration, mental confusion, and other cerebral problems of the aged. Results from the use of this drug have been remarkable.

In 1969, Denham Harman at the University of Nebraska added centrophenoxine to the feed of rats in concentrations of between 2.5 and 5 grams per kg of feed. Surprisingly, the result was an increase in mortality rate. It was interpreted that these dosages were too high, and new tests were suggested. [14]

In 1973, Richard Hochschild increased the average lifespan of aging mice by 11 per cent when he injected them with smaller dosages of centrophenoxine. In another series of experiments he commenced the injections while the mice were still young, and got even better results; between 30 and 40 per cent lifespan increases. [145] Nandy and other workers got similar results with the drug. [86] It is now clear that Harman's dosages were too high. It has since been established that in mice the $LD_{50}$ is 1,750 mg per kg of body weight orally, and 330 mg per kg intravenously. [231]

It is not yet understood precisely how centrophenoxine reduces lipofuscin deposits. Paul Gordon of Northwestern University believes that the drug, like DMAE, does not act directly upon the pigment, but instead stimulates the cell's natural scavenging abilities. [315] Roy Walford of UCLA has found that centrophenoxine, like DMAE, is also an antioxidant and free-radical deactivator. [393]

The pharmacological similarities between centrophenoxine and DMAE are not surprising. Upon entering the stomach, the drug is rapidly hydrolyzed to its components, DMAE and p-chlorophenoxyacetic acid. [127] When centrophenoxine is injected, it does not break down as quickly and may have time to accomplish its specific tasks. It would seem that oral use of centrophenoxine should offer no benefits that could not be obtained from DMAE alone, unless the presence of the acid has some unknown influence on the efficacy of DMAE.

The proper chemical name for centrophenoxine is 4-chlorophenoxyacetic acid 2-dimethylaminoethyl ester. It was first synthesized in France during the late 1950s by Rumpf and Thuillier, and was originally used as a plant-growth regulator. It is not available as a pharmaceutical in the United States, but is marketed by Lloyd-Anphar in Great Britain under the trade name Lucidryl. It is also manufactured by other companies throughout Europe under such names as Cellative, Clocete, Brenal, Helfergen, Marucotol, Methoxynal, and Proserout. Some scientists and physicians are trying to get the drug approved for use in the United States. Considering the FDA's notorious reluctance to approve foreign-made drugs, it may be a while before it is medically available here.

Although lipofuscin was officially discovered and identified in 1958, the human race has been aware of its existence for thousands of years. It most familiarly manifests itself as age pigments known as "liver spots" on the skin of older people, especially on the backs of the hands. Chapter 10 briefly discusses the ability of GH3 (European procaine) to reduce lipofuscin deposits. Several other drugs have been reported to do likewise. Chlorpromazine hydrochloride (Thorazine) changes the structure of lipofuscin so that it is more easily removed by the body's normal mechanisms, but it does not prevent the formation of lipofuscin.[323] There are some areas of the brain for which long-term administration of chlorpromazine is the only known way to reduce lipofuscin. Unfortunately, extended use of the drug shortens lifespan. Magnesium orotate and kawain have also helped control lipofuscin deposits.[100, 389] The former is the magnesium salt of orotic acid, which is now regarded as a possible B vitamin. The latter is a resinous pyrone extracted from the root of the kava-kava plant (*Piper methysticum*), which is used in the South Sea Islands as a tonic and relaxant.[357]

## Chapter Four

# Undoing the Damage

## Can Cross-Linkage
## Be Reversed?

*We can slow down the rate of cross-linkage by minimizing its causes and by the judicious use of antioxidants and free-radical deactivators. But these measures will not stop it entirely, and, most certainly, they will not reverse it. Undoing the damage is a separate problem from slowing it down or preventing it. Satisfactory solutions to this problem have not yet been found, but some interesting research is going on, and we may have some practical answers in just a few years.*

During youth, the body produces enzymes which break down cross-linked protein and preserve the supple state of the connective tissues. Scientists may soon be able to isolate and synthesize these enzymes, or restimulate their production in the aging body, or find other substances that can dissolve the irreversibly damaged collagen without unwanted side effects. Elastases, which dissolve elastin-type connective tissues, have shown some limited merit. Another group being studied are specific enzymes that dissolve old collagen in the uterus after pregnancy.

BAPN, or beta-aminopropionitrile, a chemical derived from the common chick-pea (*Lathyrus sativus*), may also be of value. BAPN does not destroy cross-linked connective tissues, but inhibits cross-linkage in newly formed elastin and collagen. During famine, the poor of India and other countries often resort to dried chick-peas as a main protein and carbohydrate staple. As a result, they sometimes suffer from a disease known as lathyrism, in which excessive amounts of BAPN result in weakened connective tissue, brittle bones, and other damage. If the correct amounts of BAPN could be administered regularly, though, they might help maintain youthful connective tissues. In 1967, Robert R. Kohn and A. M. Leash added different dosages of BAPN fumarate to the drinking water of pathogen-free CDF rats for varying lengths

$^+H_3N-CH_2CH_2CN$

*BAPN*

58

of time. Although higher dosages produced chronic lathyrism symptoms, no dosage level was found that could lengthen survival time.[182] In 1968, however, F. LaBella reported some lifespan increases in male and female rats receiving regular dosages of BAPN, as well as in those treated with another drug, semicarbazide.[203] Much more study with animals is needed before these drugs can be considered at all safe for human use, even by the most daring self-experimenting pioneers.

In 1966 at the Upjohn Company, Johan Bjorksten began a search for enzymes that can break down cross-linked protein. He uses an ingenious technique to create these enzymes. Starting with heavily cross-linked human brain tissue, he isolates the linked material by dissolving the rest of the tissues with known enzymes, and filtering out only the large, cross-linked molecules for which there are no known enzymes. He feeds this material to cultures of various microorganisms as the sole protein source. Only those that can adapt by developing a digestive enzyme for this bound protein will survive. He then isolates the enzyme and tests it on animals. If it proves to be safe, he will eventually be able to proceed with human tests. He has already had some success with a mutant strain of *Bacillus cereus*, but believes that this particular enzyme might have harmful effects on the human blood system.[23] When a safe and effective enzyme is found, we may be able to halt, and even reverse, one of the more conspicuous aspects of the aging phenomenon.

Lucien Bavetta and Marcel Nimni of the University of Southern California have given penicillamine (a modified amino acid derived from penicillin) to animals, both orally and by injection, and have noted a resultant decrease in cross-linked collagen. Experiments with human subjects are said to be in progress, but no information on their findings is available at present.[227] Penicillamine has been used as a chelating agent to treat cases of metal poisoning, and to treat Wilson's disease, a congenital, abnormal accumulation of copper in certain organs. It helps eliminate excess copper, but can also cause loss of skin tensile strength, capillary leakage, loss of leucocytes, rash, and other side effects. These symptoms can be prevented if all nutritional factors are adequate. The drug tends to deplete pyridoxine (vitamin B6) and zinc in the tissues, but daily supplements of 100 mg each of these will offset this effect. It may also deplete other trace minerals, which must also be well-supplemented. The drug, like other chelating agents, combines with metallic ions in the tissues to form metallo-amino-acid complexes. These are easily removed from the tissues by excretion.

The preferred form of the drug is D-acetylpenicillamine, which is the least toxic, most stable, and most readily absorbed by mouth. The D form does not induce pyridoxine deficiency, and the acetyl portion protects the amino group from degradation.[55] It is produced by Merck, Sharp, and Dohme, and is available by

$$COO^-$$
$$|$$
$$^+H_3N - CH$$
$$|$$
$$HS - C - CH_3$$
$$|$$
$$CH_3$$

*Penicillamine*

prescription. The medicinal dosage is 250 mg daily, increasing to 250 to 500 mg four times daily, by mouth. This is probably more than is necessary for the dissolution of cross-linked protein, especially when it is taken on a lifelong basis. An additional danger with this drug is that prolonged use can result in immunity to the antibiotic effects of penicillin.

At present, no available drug can safely and certainly reverse accumulations of cross-linked protein, although researchers anticipate a major breakthrough within the next five years. Meanwhile, the best that self-experimenters can do is minimize the frequency of damaging cross-linkages by using safe antioxidants and avoiding excessive amounts of polyunsaturated fatty acids, rancid foods, stress, toxic substances, and other proliferators of free radicals and lipid peroxidation. If diet and exercise are also adequate, health should be good, and the body will continue to produce ample quantities of its own protective enzymes for as many years as possible.

# Chapter Five

# Promoting Regeneration

## Nucleic Acids and Protein Regeneration

*The human body has a remarkable capacity for regeneration. Damaged DNA can be repaired, and the body tends to remove and replace misconstructed proteins. How can we assist these natural processes? There are several things that can be done, and thousands of people are already doing some of them.*

In Chapter 2 we saw briefly that the by-products of lipid peroxidation can react with DNA and RNA, and can disrupt their genetic information so much that they synthesize abnormal protein. Precisely how this happens is not fully understood. Johan Bjorksten believes that cross-linkages are formed between portions of the DNA's spiral helices. Richard Kohn and others think that cross-linkages occur only in the connective tissues, and never touch anything within the cell, much less the nucleus. The evidence, however, is beginning to accrue in favor of Bjorksten's view. His opponents argue that cross-links can only take place between proteins or proteinaceous substances, such as enzymes. Proponents of Bjorksten's hypothesis point out that the chromosomes are actually nucleoproteins, that is, protein and nucleic-acid combinations. There is much evidence that disruptions of genetic data do occur with age, and result in an increase of missynthesized proteins. It is known that RNA levels decrease after the age of forty, and there is evidence that RNA's resistance to misprogramming weakens with age. [14, 258] Reduction of protein and enzyme formation in later years may be due to these changes.

It is also known that histones tend to cling to DNA in old age, and probably cause errors in transmission of genetic information to the RNA. Histones are types of water-soluble nucleoproteins that appear to play a role in gene repression.

The double-stranded DNA structure within each cell contains all the genetic information for every organ of the body. Not all of that information, however, is needed or even wanted by any given cell. A skin cell, for example, contains all the information for constructing the individual's skin. It also contains information for constructing his eyes, his liver, his hair, and every other organ of his body. Clearly, all this information cannot be expressed in every cell of the body, or biological chaos would prevail. Furthermore, some cells must express different information at different times in the life cycle of the individual. To confine the genetic information in a cell to that which is pertinent at the time, histones cover up all unwanted information, preventing its transcription to the messenger RNA. When histone-blocked information is needed, other nucleoproteins known as nonhistones remove the histones from the desired gene site. Excessive histone accumulation and lack of the activated nonhistones needed to remove them can slow down or confound DNA/RNA protein synthesis, and may be contributing causes of the aging process.

Recent research has asked whether histones might be able to switch genes on as well as off, since DNA and histones were found bound tightly (but reversibly) to each other. However, information on the makeup of histones from various organisms (both plants and animals) shows that the structure has changed very little with evolution. So, although DNA can't be copied while it is bound to histones, the actual switching on of the genes is probably carried out by other, unidentified specialized molecules. Histones, then, may function to "wrap up" the DNA in a tight package when it isn't being used.

Missynthesized proteins cause damage in several ways. They are larger than normal proteins and compete with them for nutrients. They take up space and crowd out the normal constituents of the cells. They deluge the cells with waste materials, which results in cellular toxification and strangulation. Because they are defective, the body must produce more proteins to replace them. This is a drain on energies and material resources. If the correct protein is not synthesized, either that protein's function will not be carried out, or a defective protein will replace the missing one and the function of the structure or enzyme will be altered or impaired. When the immunologic system recognizes these proteins as abnormal (see Chapter 7) and attacks them, it is distracted from its main task of defending the body from invaders. It is also an additional energy drain.

To cope with the problems of altered DNA or RNA, we must prevent lipid peroxidation and free-radical reactions within the cell, assist the repair of the genetic coding in the DNA, and abet the decomposition of the missynthesized proteins, so that they can be replaced by correctly formed ones. We have already discussed various ways to prevent or minimize lipid peroxidation and free-radical damage by avoiding their causes and by obtaining sufficient antioxidants and free-radical deactivators in the diet.

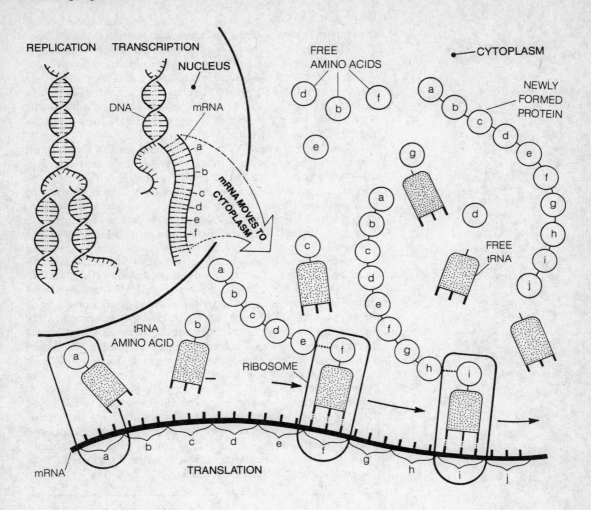

REPLICATION    TRANSCRIPTION

NUCLEUS

FREE AMINO ACIDS

CYTOPLASM

DNA    mRNA

NEWLY FORMED PROTEIN

mRNA MOVES TO CYTOPLASM

FREE tRNA

tRNA AMINO ACID

RIBOSOME

mRNA    TRANSLATION

*Protein synthesis and missynthesis.*

The DNA is the molecule which stores the original information for the composition of each protein. It duplicates itself in a process called *replication*. In *transcription* the information for the required protein(s) is copied onto a strand of mRNA (messenger RNA). The mRNA moves from the nucleus to the cytoplasm, where it is *translated* into a sequence of amino acids. Each group of three "letters" (bases) in the RNA represents one specific amino acid. The amino acids are brought to the point of translation (the ribosome) by a tRNA (transfer RNA; the ribosome actually takes two tRNAs at a time), which matches its three letters to the correct three letters on the mRNA. The correct amino acid is joined to the chain of amino acids which make up the new protein; the ribosome then slides to the next three-letter "word," and the process is repeated until the protein is completed.

Missynthesis occurs when an error happens in any one of these matchings or transfers—in either the replication, the transcription, or the translation. For example, if in the making of the mRNA, one of the DNA bases is misread, then the protein made on that mRNA would probably have a different amino acid at that position. This would cause all the protein made on that mRNA to be defective.

The radioprotectant properties of rutins and other substances are also important in preventing lipid peroxidation and DNA damage.

Damaged DNA has a tendency to return to normal if the disruption is not too severe or too long perpetuated. If a portion of one strand of the DNA's double helix is altered, the corresponding portion of the other strand supplies the information needed to make the correction. A youthful condition of the cells favors this repair. The older the cells become, the more difficult it is for altered DNA to right itself.

Various nutritional factors are required for DNA repair and correct protein synthesis. Among these are the essential amino acids, ascorbic acid, and the B vitamins — especially biotin, pantothenic acid, and pyridoxine ($B_6$) — which assist in the formation of nucleotides. Choline is needed for the synthesis of nucleic acids. Folic acid, riboflavin, zinc, manganese, and chromium are necessary for cell division and the production of DNA and RNA. [105, 258] Orotic acid is also of value, since it is a precursor of the pyrimidines, from which nucleotides and nucleosides are constructed. These, in turn, are incorporated into the structures of DNA and RNA. Several reports indicate that sulfur amino acids, seleno-amino acids, ascorbic acid, and vitamin E, combined, promote DNA and RNA repair. [258] No doubt, scientists will eventually discover that many other vitamins and minerals play key roles in DNA/RNA repair and maintenance. If you are following a sound basic nutrition program, such as the one outlined in Chapter 6, you will already be getting all you need of these substances.

Fortunately, missynthesized proteins are not integrated into the cells as rapidly as normal proteins. They are therefore exposed for some while to the action of the body's immunological defense system, which attacks these foreign-seeming proteins and breaks them down into raw materials, which can be used to synthesize protein, this time correctly, one hopes.

---

Protein synthesis, like all biological activities, requires energy. Decreased RNA in the cells of persons over forty causes protein synthesis to place a greater burden upon the cells. Adequate nutrition and rest are as necessary for adults as they are for growing children. Moderate exercise stimulates cell division and protein formation. It also keeps the toxic by-products of all this activity moving through the channels of excretion.

---

Nucleic acids are also essential in the formation of DNA and RNA, although there is some controversy about whether they must be obtained dietetically. Some writings on health and life extension recommend occasional, brief diets that are high in nucleic acids, or regular supplements of nucleic acids, coordinated with a program of abundant vitamins, minerals, and amino acids to promote the repair of damaged DNA and RNA and to encourage the synthesis of correctly formed protein. A typical program might involve taking 1,000 to 2,000 mg of nucleic acids daily for three weeks out of every three or four months, and staying on a low or moderate intake the rest of the time. [194] However, since DNA/RNA repair and protein synthesis are continuous processes, I believe it is better to supply the body regularly with the nucleic acids and other materials required for these activities. There may be some increased protein synthesis after illness, because the body produces biostimulants at such times. A convalescing person might consider engaging in a brief program of increased amino acids, nucleic acids, vitamins, and minerals.

The main reason for the break of several months between treatments is that nucleic acids metabolize into purines, which in turn form uric acid. Although uric acid is a normal metabolite in the body, excessive amounts of it can be harmful to the cells. When there is both excessive uric acid and excessive sodium in the system, the two combine to cause gout. The tendency toward this disease is due to a genetic deficiency in the enzyme that converts certain purine bases to nucleotides, or to a defect in feedback-control mechanisms involved in purine synthesis. Except for individuals who are thus inclined toward gout, the fear that dietary nucleic acids can cause dangerous rises in uric acid appears to have been exaggerated. The amounts of uric acid formed because of stress, overwork, shock, alcohol excesses, suppressed anger, exposure to cold, and extended fasts far exceed those that might result from a nucleic-acid-rich diet. [87, 333] Furthermore, much can be done to keep amounts of uric acid low.

The conventional biochemical view is that, in humans, uric acid (as urate) is the final product of purine degradation. However, Adelle Davis discusses the gout and uric-acid problem at length in her popular book *Let's Get Well,* and she disagrees. [76] She points out that pantothenic acid (vitamin B5) converts uric acid to ammonia and urea, which are easily excreted. [302, 359] Thiamine (B1) also helps keep the amounts of uric acid down. [18, 37, 391] All antistress vitamins and minerals (B vitamins, ascorbic acid, calcium, and magnesium) help prevent stress-induced rises in uric acid. Ascorbic acid also assists in the excretion of this and other toxins. Vitamins A and E, along with moderate but adequate amounts of essential polyunsaturated fatty acids, also help protect the cells from uric-acid damage. Improperly balanced protein can increase uric-acid production, especially if the diet is high in glycine (an amino acid abundant in gelatin). [15, 245] If incomplete protein foods, such as corn, beans, or lentils are eaten, they should be balanced *at the same meal* with complete protein foods (meat, cheese, milk, eggs, seafoods, etc.) or complementary protein sources, such as whole grains. Stress avoidance, regular exercise, adequate sleep, and a high liquid intake are very important in keeping amounts of uric acid down. At least four glasses of water and several glasses of milk, fruit juices, and vegetable juices taken daily will assist in the dissolution and excretion of uric acid. The juices also help maintain an alkaline condition, which keeps the uric acid in solution to facilitate excretion. Intestinal bacteria (acidophilus) utilize uric acid, and thereby help get rid of it. [345]

All these ways of minimizing uric acid will take place automatically in any sound nutritional program. If you are meeting all your nutritional requirements, maintaining healthy intestinal flora, avoiding undue stress and toxic drugs (alcohol, caffeine, nicotine, etc.), and getting proper exercise and rest, in short, if you are living right, you should be able to include 1,000 to 2,000 mg of nucleic acids in your daily diet without concern about rises in uric acid. This much nucleic acid can be furnished by a fairly ordinary diet.

The major argument against diets high in nucleic acids and DNA/RNA supplements is not that they might increase uric acid, but that they are not needed in the diet, because the body can synthesize them from proteins and carbohydrates. Dr. Benjamin Frank, a leading nucleic-acid expert and author of several books on the subject, counters this argument by pointing out that there are enzymes in the gastrointestinal tract (nucleases) that break down nucleic acids into nucleotides, and biosynthetic pathways in our cells for converting these nucleotides back into nucleic acids. Since nucleic acids are so plentiful in our foods, it appears that nature intends us to obtain at least some of them dietetically.

In his popular book *Dr. Frank's No-Aging Diet*, Dr. Frank recommends a daily intake of 1,000 to 2,000 mg of nucleic acids, obtained by eating foods that are rich in them. He reports that after about two months on this regimen, one will notice improvements in strength, energy, physical appearance, and general health. Wrinkles and deep facial lines begin to disappear. The skin becomes moist and glowing, because of improved cell function and increased production of hyaluronic acid, the skin's moisture-retention factor, which usually diminishes with age. Age pigments in the skin gradually fade. There is an increased regrowth of hair on the scalp, and sometimes a return of pigmentation to graying hair.

Earlier, we spoke of the tiny organelles within the cell known as the mitochondria. These granular bodies are the powerhouses of the cell. Within them adenosine triphosphate (ATP), the basic fuel of life, is manufactured and expended. ATP is a nucleotide, and can be synthesized from nucleic acids. This is the chief reason that Dr. Frank's diet augments energy and strength. Increased ATP also results in more efficient use of oxygen, which means less lipid peroxidation.

The mainstay of Dr. Frank's diet is sardines, eaten four times a week. Besides being one of the richest sources of nucleic acids, they are an excellent source of selenium and other trace minerals. They contain substantial amounts of DMAE, the antioxidant and precursor substance that is converted to choline and acetylcholine in the brain. Sardines and other seafood are high in protein and essential fatty acids, and low in cholesterol. They also have high levels of xanthine, a purine from which the body can manufacture guanosine diphosphate, which is required for metabolic efficiency. Because they are small fish and therefore on the bottom of the food chain, they contain lower concentrations of pollutants than the larger, fish-eating fish. Whether it is necessary or not to obtain nucleic acids dietetically, there is much to be gained from sardines and other foods suggested in Dr. Frank's diet. [103, 104, 105]

As far back as 1928, longevity experiments have been carried out with nucleic acids. At that time, T. B. Robertson, in Australia, fed 25 mg of yeast-derived nucleic acids daily to white mice, starting after weaning and continuing until death. The result was a 16 per cent increase in lifespan. [304] Proportionately, for a 150-pound human, this amount would equal about 70

## Approximate Nucleic-Acid Content of Foods [a]

| FOOD SOURCE | NUCLEIC ACIDS [b] | FOOD SOURCE | NUCLEIC ACIDS [b] |
|---|---|---|---|
| Brewer's yeast | 5,000 [c] | Baby lima beans [d] | 200 |
| Sardines (small, canned) | 600 | Chicken heart | 175 |
| Pinto beans [d] | 475 | Split peas [d] | 175 |
| Lentils [d] | 475 | Red beans [d] | 150 |
| Chicken liver | 400 | Beef kidney | 125 |
| Garbanzo beans [d] | 350 | Mackerel (canned) | 125 |
| Anchovies (fresh) | 350 | Squid (fresh) | 100 |
| Blackeye peas [d] | 300 | Lamb liver | 100 |
| Small white beans [d] | 300 | Clams (fresh) | 75 |
| Lima beans (large) [d] | 300 | Herring (canned) | 75 |
| Salmon (fresh) | 300 | Beef brain | 50 |
| Great northern beans [d] | 275 | Lamb or beef heart | 50 |
| Cranberry beans [d] | 250 | Clams (canned) | 50 |
| Beef or pork liver | 250 | Salmon (canned) | 25 |
| Oysters (canned) | 250 | Most muscle meats | 25 |
| Mackerel (fresh) | 200 | | |

[a] Most of this information is derived from *Dr. Frank's No-Aging Diet*, p. 104, and rounded off to multiples of 25 mg. The data was supplied to Dr. Benjamin S. Frank by Dr. A. J. Clifford, Professor of Nutrition at the University of California, Davis.

[b] Expressed as mg per 100 grams (3.5 oz.) of the food source.

[c] Different brands range between 2,500 and 8,000 mg, or 175 to 550 mg per tablespoonful (7 grams). Read the label.

[d] All legumes as 100 grams dried weight.

grams (2.5 ounces). Normally, senescent weight loss occurs in these animals after their seventieth week of life, but it was delayed in the treated animals. In 1946, T. S. Gardner began feeding 2.5 mg of yeast-derived nucleic acids daily to albino mice when they were 600 days old and on the brink of old age. They retained their vigor and vitality longer than the controls, had less tendency toward senile blindness, and averaged a 9 per cent increase in lifespan. In general, the treated mice were healthier and more active than the controls, and, unlike the controls, did not exhibit any significant weight loss before death.[113] For a 150-pound human, the equivalent dose would be about 7,000 mg (a quarter ounce).

More recently, Hans J. Kugler injected Snell-Bagg dwarf mice with organ-derived nucleic acids and more than doubled their usual lifespans of three to five months.[197] The product used by Kugler was Regeneresen, also known as RN-13, which contains RNA from twelve different organs: placenta, testes, ovaries, hypothalamus, adrenal cortices, pituitary, thalamus, spleen, vascular walls, cerebral cortex, liver, and kidneys, plus yeast-derived nucleic acid. RN-13 injections are available from some rejuvenation doctors in Germany and other European countries. The combination is said to normalize protein synthesis in all organs represented, and to have a generally beneficial influence on the entire body. Learning, memory, and general brain function are also improved by this substance. The basic principle of Regeneresen therapy is that when RNA from a specific organ is injected intramuscularly, it benefits mainly the same organ of the recipient. For this reason, RN-13 and similar products are also known as organ-specific nucleic acids. It does not matter that the organs are from a different species than the recipient. This principle is also involved in the technique known as cell therapy (see Chapter 11).

Kugler and others believe that combined yeast-derived and organ-specific nucleic acids have greater life-extending value than yeast-derived nucleic acids alone.[196] Outstanding results have been obtained, however, by Dr. Max Wolf, a Viennese living in Manhattan, with a mutated yeast which he calls "yeast meat." The yeast cells are mutated with ultraviolet light and grown on a special protein culture medium. Most nutritional yeasts sold in health-food stores contain 20 to 50 per cent protein. Wolf's product contains 70 to 80 per cent, and is also extra rich in B vitamins. Rats fed yeast meat as their sole source of protein doubled their normal lifespans. Wolf has been able to produce the yeast at a cost of about 20 cents a pound. By varying the glutamic-acid content, he can alter the flavor to resemble that of different meats, such as chicken, pork, beef, and veal.[225] As meat becomes more and more expensive, it may be replaced by new and better protein foods like Max Wolf's yeast meat, and, as a fringe benefit, we may all enjoy longer and healthier lives.

# Chapter Six
# Nutrition and Aging

*We all know that vitamins and minerals are good for us. Most of us have some vague understanding of what a few of these nutrients do, but beyond that there is usually a vast gap of ignorance. Our lack of knowledge, however, doesn't stop us from spending over a billion dollars annually on vitamin pills. Most of us don't even know how to use nutritional supplements effectively. No wonder they rarely fulfill our expectations!*

*Nutrition is a fairly complex study. No single vitamin or mineral functions entirely on its own; each interacts and works in harmony with all the others. Books that try to unravel the complexity and explain this mutual dependence often deluge the reader with data and leave him more confused than ever.*

*Although this chapter primarily concerns the relationships between nutrition and longevity, it touches on the general functions of the various vitamins and minerals. Perhaps, because of its brevity, it will give the reader a concise grasp of the subject.*

In a sense, any vitamin, mineral, or other nutritional factor may be regarded as an anti-aging drug. Deprive the body of an essential nutrient, and it will age more rapidly and die prematurely. Give the body all it needs, and the probabilities of good health and long life are greatly increased. Still, as we have already seen, some nutritional components do play special roles in the control of aging. In large-enough dosages, they have protective and therapeutic properties, distinct from their usual nutritional functions. But these meganutrients and other life-extension drugs cannot give the desired results unless all nutritional requirements are met. This brief chapter cannot cover the subject of total nutrition. Many other books are available that cover it quite well. But we do need to consider some nutritional materials, not yet discussed, that contribute in special ways to maintaining youthful vigor and delaying aging. For the most part, we will only consider aspects of these substances that concern the control of aging, or of age-related problems.

## Vitamins

We mentioned earlier that vitamin E helps prevent the oxidation of vitamin A. The latter, however, is also a powerful antioxidant and free-radical deactivator. During the 1940s, Henry Sherman at Columbia University extended the lifespans of male Osborne-Mendel rats by 10 per cent, and of females by 20 per cent, by giving them supplemental dosages of vitamin A.[341, 342] The vitamin also helps decrease cholesterol. For a period of ten years, two Australian physicians gave extra dosages of vitamins A and D to a group of patients. At the end of this period, the treated patients had about a third less cholesterol than the untreated ones.[316] Vitamin D can serve as an antistress agent, because it maintains good amounts of calcium, which has a calming effect, in the blood. It also helps the bones retain calcium, and can prevent osteoporosis and related problems in the aged and in postmenopausal women. The optimal adult dosage for vitamin A is usually around 30,000 I.U. daily (10,000 with each meal); for vitamin D, about 5,000 I.U. daily (also in divided doses). Megadosages of these vitamins should not be taken. Dangerous side effects can develop after several month's daily use of 50,000 to 100,000 I.U. of vitamin A, or more than 25,000 I.U. of vitamin D. Prolonged overdosage of vitamin A can cause rupturing of lysosome membranes, which could accelerate the aging process. Adequate amounts of magnesium, choline, and vitamins C and E in the diet can help prevent overdosage reactions to A and D. Vitamins A and D, like vitamin E, are oil-soluble, and are best assimilated when taken together at meals.[62, 69, 83]

The B vitamins also combat the effects of stress, especially when taken in combination. Pantothenic acid (vitamin B5) is the most outstanding in this respect. Roger J. Williams, its discoverer, found it to be the substance in royal jelly that extends the life of the queen bee far beyond that of the worker. After several experiments showed that it also lengthened the lives of fruit flies, Pelton and Williams at the University of Texas gave 300 mcg of the vitamin daily to male and female C-57 black mice, and increased their lifespans by about 20 per cent.[265] This dosage, 12 mg per kg of body weight, would proportionally equal 840 mg for a 150-pound human. Although pantothenic acid has been used successfully to relieve arthritis, large dosages have been reported to increase sensitivity painfully to minor dental caries and arthritic joints.[74, 276] Yet this vitamin is essential for maintaining calcium in the bones and teeth. Except for rare cases of minor side effects, 10,000 mg or more has been found to be a safe

"At best the RDAs are only a 'recommended' allowance at antediluvian levels designed to prevent some terrible disease. At worst they are based on conflicts of interest and self-serving views of certain portions of the food industry. Almost never are they provided at levels to provide for optimum health and nutrition."

Senator William Proxmire, *Let's Live* (1974)

"Often doctors are trained in nutrition by doctors who heard it from another doctor who made it up."

Dr. Julian B. Schorr, New York Blood Center, *Wall Street Journal* (Jan. 1971)

dosage.[301] The RDA for pantothenic acid is 10 to 15 mg a day. Most modern nutritionists recommend at least 100 mg daily, and much more while under stress. Some recommend that 200 to 400 mg be taken three times a day. You should be able to find your ideal daily dosage by trial and observation, somewhere between 100 and 1,200 mg. Pantothenic acid is also a constituent of coenzyme A, which is involved in the transfer of acetyl groups. This acetylation is essential for energy metabolism, antibody formation, and the synthesis of acetylcholine in the brain and nervous system.[58, 276] There have been reports of gray hair returning to its original color when 300 mg each of pantothenic acid and PABA were taken daily in combination with 5 mg of folic acid and adequate amounts of the other B vitamins.[63, 75] Because they are required to metabolize pantothenic acid, 1 mg of folic acid and 100 mg of biotin should be taken with every 300 mg of that vitamin.

Folic acid also plays a key role in cell division, the production of DNA and RNA, and correct protein synthesis. A deficiency of the vitamin can lead to hair loss. Baldness in men is often caused by unusually high individual requirements for this and other B vitamins that are not being fulfilled. Regrowth of hair often occurs when the anti-graying combination is taken along with 1,500 mg of inositol, 50 to 100 mg of vitamin B6, and an otherwise healthy, protein-rich diet.[171]

Vitamin B6 (pyridoxine) is another important antistress agent. It is also needed for correct protein synthesis, to properly metabolize fats in the diet, and thus to help prevent cholesterol accumulation. Combined with zinc, it can help relieve edema during menopause. Under special stress situations, the normal 50 to 100 mg dosage can be increased to 500 mg.[64, 116, 243, 275]

PABA (para-aminobenzoic acid) is a B vitamin that belongs to the group of substances known as aromatic amines. These materials have some antioxidant activity. PABA protects laboratory animals exposed to ozone.[121] It is also an antistress factor and an anti-graying agent. It is often used as a sunscreen in suntan lotions. It does not block the beneficial, tanning rays of the sun, but screens out the damaging portions of the ultraviolet spectrum, which are a major cause of premature skin wrinkling.[413] It is reported that PABA's solar-protective properties also work when it is taken internally. A daily intake of 1,000 mg has enabled fair-skinned people to tolerate as much sun as dark-skinned people.[63] This amount is a good basic dosage, and 3,000 mg or more can be taken during stress or exposure to ozone. PABA interferes with the antibiotic activity of sulfa drugs, and must not be taken when these are prescribed; but substantial amounts of PABA should be taken after treatment, since the sulfa drugs will produce a deficiency of it. If sulfadiazine is used regularly as a life-extension agent (see page 139), PABA should be supple-

COO⁻

NH₂

*PABA*

✓

$$HOCH_2CH_2-\overset{\overset{\displaystyle CH_3}{|}}{\underset{\underset{\displaystyle CH_3}{|}}{N^+}}-CH_3$$

*Choline*

see p 56

✓

$$CH_3C\overset{\displaystyle O}{\underset{\displaystyle OCH_2CH_2}{{=}}}-\overset{\overset{\displaystyle CH_3}{|}}{\underset{\underset{\displaystyle CH_3}{|}}{N^+}}-CH_3$$

*Acetylcholine*

The neurotransmitter acetylcholine is made from choline and acetate. Lecithin is a good source of choline.

mented. In the body, procaine breaks down to PABA and DEAE (see Chapter 10).

Choline is not always regarded as a vitamin, because it can be manufactured in the body from methionine, folic acid, and vitamin B12.[63] However, since our real choline needs are quite high, and since methionine is needed for protein building, detoxification, and free-radical deactivation, it is better to provide the choline than to tax the methionine supplies. Combined with inositol, choline helps to reduce cholesterol levels.[202] Soy lecithin, sold in health-food stores, is rich in both substances. A daily dosage of 1,000 mg of each of these vitamins—up to 3,000 mg if fat intake is high—is recommended. From choline, the body synthesizes acetylcholine, which is essential for brain function. DMAE, one of the antioxidants discussed in Chapter 2, reaches the brain and is converted to choline and acetylcholine. Inositol concentrates in the heart muscle and eye lens, and apparently helps maintain normal heart function and vision.

Vitamin B1 (thiamine) is needed to convert sugars to caloric energy. The RDA is 1 mg, but more is usually needed. Individual requirements vary, but between 25 and 100 mg is usually adequate.[257] More can be taken during periods of stress, and 500 to 1,000 mg can give a lift when energies are low. There is some danger that the prolonged use of thiamine in these stimulant dosages may disrupt the normal B balance, causing deficiencies of other B vitamins, although this is less of a problem if the others are well supplied. If chronic exhaustion is a persistent problem, you should try to find the cause, rather than abuse the vitamin. Massive dosages of up to 4,000 mg of B1 along with other vitamins have been used successfully to treat some of the symptoms of chronic alcoholism. This therapy should be supervised by a physician. There have been reports that thiamine exhibits some antioxidant activity, possibly because of the sulfur in its structure.[127, 128] Its main value in protecting against oxidation, though, is that it regulates and normalizes oxidative metabolism by means of its role in transforming glucose to energy.[239]

Vitamin B2 (riboflavin) is another important antistress factor. Prolonged deficiency can result in wrinkles about the mouth, commonly known as whistle marks. These are usually associated with aging in women, but can happen at any age, and to either sex. When the vitamin is adequately supplied along with linoleic acid, folic acid, pantothenic acid, and vitamin B6, these lines gradually disappear.[66] The RDA of less than 2 mg is far below the ideal dosage, which is more in the vicinity of 50 to 100 mg normally, and two or three times this during stress. Since vitamins B2 and B6 tend to deplete each other during their normal metabolism, dosages of these two should be kept fairly equal.

Vitamin B3 (niacin) also protects against stress. It is involved in protein and carbohydrate metabolism and in the formation of certain enzymes associates with mental health. It also helps prevent many aging symptoms. It reduces fatty deposits in the skin and cholesterol accumulations in the arteries. [40, 99] It counteracts blood clotting, a frequent cause of premature death, stroke, heart attack, and loss of normal brain functioning. It also breaks up sludging of the red corpuscles. The vitamin places a negative charge on the surface of red blood-cell membranes, which further improves their oxygen-carrying ability. [242] It also regresses atherosclerosis and improves circulation. [358] As far back as 1938, it had been known that niacin can normalize an abnormal electrocardiogram. [352] The RDA for niacin is about 20 mg, but this is merely the amount some people need to avoid pellagra, the extreme deficiency syndrome. The actual individual requirements for this vitamin vary more widely than for other vitamins. Abram Hoffer and Humphrey Osmond found that massive dosages of B3 can prevent and control certain types of schizophrenia, and that some patients need as much as 18,000 mg daily. [148, 149] These huge dosages, however, should only be taken under the supervision of a qualified physician and as an adjuvant to psychotherapy. There have been reports of serious side effects from megadosages of niacin, including ulcers, jaundice, liver damage, male sexual impotence, colitis, and diabetes-like symptoms. They seem to be due to individual sensitivity, and can usually be avoided if 1,000 mg of vitamin C and 100 mg each of B1 and B6 are taken with every 1,000 mg of niacin. Normally, even moderately large doses of niacin will cause a harmless flushing and tingling of the skin, because it releases histamines from the basal cells. This effect can be minimized if one takes two aspirins or one antihistamine tablet an hour before taking the niacin. Niacinamide, another form of the vitamin, does not cause this reaction, but may cause depression in some individuals. A regular dosage of 200 to 500 mg of vitamin B3 can be taken three times daily under normal conditions. During stress, the dosage can be increased to 1,000 mg, three times a day. These dosages are within the margins of safety, especially if other nutritional factors are in order. It is only when daily dosages exceeding 5,000 mg are continued for periods longer than two months that medical supervision is suggested. [65, 138, 240, 257]

Vitamin B12 (cobalamine) is also effective in combatting stress and fatigue. It is an essential growth factor, necessary for the synthesis of nucleic acids and nucleoproteins, and for proper maintenance of the brain and nerves. Inadequate levels of this vitamin have been associated with late-onset schizophrenia and some forms of senile dementia. [271] Although less than 3 mcg daily is needed to prevent extreme deficiency symptoms (pernicious anemia and nerve degeneration), many people, especially total vegetarians, fail to get even that amount. For one thing, it is rarely if ever found in foods from the plant kingdom, and then only in insignificant traces. Also, a particular mucoprotein is needed to facilitate absorption of it. This substance, known as the

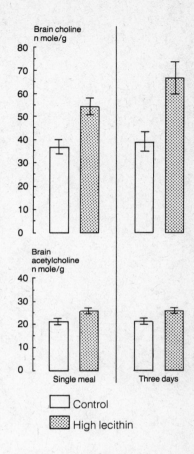

*Lecithin consumption and acetylcholine in the brain.*

Can the amount of lecithin eaten affect the amounts of choline and acetylcholine in the tissues where they act? When rats were fed lecithin granules (10 to 20 per cent pure lecithin) as 50 per cent of their diet, an increase in brain choline and acetylcholine concentrations were found after one meal. The increase was even more pronounced after three days of feeding. This suggests that the concentration of something as central as a neurotransmitter (acetylcholine) is under direct nutritional control.

B12 intrinsic factor, is secreted in the stomach by the parietal cells of the gastric mucosa. As we age, less of it is produced. One reason for this is that autoimmune reactions, which increase with age (see Chapter 7), are often directed against these cells. [114] The vitamin is frequently sold in tablet form with the intrinsic factor added. Large amounts of the vitamin can alleviate exhaustion, increase energy, correct fatigue-induced impotence, and relieve the mental symptoms of deficiency. Only a small percentage of large oral doses can be assimilated, however. The only way to derive the full value of large dosages is through injection. The injectable vitamin is produced by several pharmaceutical companies in ampules of 1 cc., containing 500 mcg. Individual dosages range between 500 and 3,000 mcg every 3 to 7 days. The usual form of the vitamin is cyanocobalamin, but this may be toxic to some individuals. In 1970, researchers in England found optic nerve damage in patients sensitive to the cyano portion of the vitamin. The safer form of this vitamin for cyano-sensitive individuals is hydroxocobalamine (B12b), which also gives serum levels that are higher and last three times longer. [101] Because the oral dosage is small and is broken down to the hydroxo form during assimilation, tablets of cyanocobalamin present no problem to cyano-sensitive persons. Some companies sell B12 tablets in dosages as high as 200 mcg. The only advantage of these is that, in dosages exceeding 25 mcg, a small percentage of the vitamin may be absorbed, even without the intrinsic factor. If the body is not producing enough of this factor, it is better to take lower-dosage tablets that also contain the intrinsic factor, or to receive occasional injections. [241]

Vitamin B15 (pangamic acid) prevents oxygen starvation in the tissues by stimulating normal oxidative metabolism. At the same time, it reduces random oxidation in the cells, and is therefore valuable in the control of aging. It detoxifies the body by stimulating the hypophyseal-adrenal system, lowers cholesterols, prevents fatty degeneration of the liver, regulates the use of glucose, and improves the metabolism of protein in the heart. [185] Despite these and many other virtues, the medical establishment in this country has ignored this vitamin. Even most popular nutrition authors have failed to mention it. Although it is nontoxic, California and some other states forbid its sale. Still, some health-food stores in California will sell it under the counter to known customers. It is perfectly legal for individuals to mail-order it from out of state (see Appendix A). The ideal dosage seems to be around 50 milligrams 3 to 5 times a day.

Vitamin B17 (amygdalin, also called laetrile) is another natural substance that has been suppressed by the medical establishment and outlawed by the government, mainly because of claims that it can control cancer. Proponents say that it is a vitamin, not a medicine, and that cancer may develop when there is a deficiency. It is also reported to help prevent other degenerative diseases of aging, including hardening of the arteries and cirrhosis of the liver. It is said to be most effective when taken with a diet rich in sulfur amino acids, such as cysteine and methionine. [179] Fair amounts of amygdalin are found in various seeds, sprouts, legumes, nuts, berries, grains, and cabbage-like vegetables, but apricot kernels are by far the richest source. [384] Since the FDA has outlawed the sale of this vitamin, it must be obtained from nature. The recommended daily dosage range is between 200 and 800 mg. Seven apricot kernels can supply about 100 mg. The kernels should be taken in divided dosages, with meals. They must be chewed thoroughly, or ground up and put in capsules. There have been instances of brief dizziness and nausea from single doses of amygdalin exceeding 1,000 mg.

Vitamin F is a name sometimes used for the three essential polyunsaturated fatty acids (PUFAs): linoleic, linolenic, and arachidonic acids. These are found in seeds, nuts, legumes, and fish; to some extent in meats, egg yolks, and dairy fats; and especially in oils of safflower, corn, wheat germ, soybean, sesame, cottonseed, and peanut. Olive oil is fairly low in PUFAs, and coconut oil contains none. During the past twenty years or so, polyunsaturated oils have become popular because they help to lower cholesterol levels in the blood. Although it has also been found that excessive intake of PUFAs can increase the incidence of cancer and hasten aging, [136, 255, 339] the polyunsaturate craze still continues. PUFAs contribute to cancer and aging because they tend to react rapidly with oxygen to form lipid peroxides and free radicals. Furthermore, there is evidence that cholesterol removed from the blood by high-PUFA diets is transferred to the tissues, where it can increase membrane damage.

Small amounts of polyunsaturated oils can be used in salads safely and beneficially, particularly if adequate supplies of vitamin E and other antioxidants are included in the diet. Adding antioxidants to oils, as described in Chapter 2, slows the rate of oxidation. Polyunsaturated oils should be stored in the refrigerator. It is better to buy only small bottles, so that the oil is not kept for very long. Polyunsaturated oils should not be used for cooking. Heating them to 200°F or higher causes chemical changes that can increase the incidence of atherosclerosis. Coconut oil is better for cooking.

Unrefined oils that are high in PUFAs are usually also fairly rich in lecithin, the common name for the chemical phosphatidal choline. The vegetable lecithin extracted from soy oil and sold in health-food stores is a mixture of phosphatidal choline and other, related compounds. It is a very useful antiaging superfood in that it helps dissolve cholesterol accumulations [2, 189] and is somewhat an antioxidant. [268, 406] The phospholipids are essential for cell and organelle membranes. One or two tablespoonfuls of soy lecithin can be taken daily, preferably with meals and oil-soluble vitamins. It has a mild vegetable-like taste that does not much affect

"If a person is particular about the quality of wine he drinks, he's a connoisseur. If he's particular about the quality of food he eats, he's a nut."

William Dufty,
author of *Sugar Blues*

the flavor of foods or blender drinks to which it is added. It is available in both liquid and granule form; capsules are not economical.

## Minerals

Some minerals, such as calcium and magnesium, are required in fairly large quantities; others, only in traces. The importance of many of these trace minerals is often ignored. It is frequently assumed that we obtain enough of them through our foods, but the soils in some areas are almost totally lacking in many of these elements. Furthermore, vegetables grown in heavily nitrated soils do not take up these minerals too well. As was mentioned in the section on selenium, some minerals may be toxic in amounts only a few times higher than the optimal dosage. The toxicity is often due to the form in which the mineral is taken and the manner in which it is stored in the tissues.

Chelated minerals are usually recommended for nutritional use, because they are assimilated up to ten times better than nonchelated ones. In terms of nutrition, chelated means that the mineral is molecularly bound in a complex with amino acids. In a healthy person, nonchelated minerals are chelated in the stomach during digestion. But if digestion is poor, chelated minerals should be taken. They are available at all health-food stores.

Sodium and potassium are required in fairly substantial amounts, but are so abundant in nature that there is usually no problem obtaining them. The main concern is to maintain a balance of the two elements, which tend to displace each other in the tissues. Sodium causes the tissues to retain water, whereas potassium expels it. Most of us get more sodium than we need from salt, MSG (monosodium glutamate), and "hidden" sodium in commercially prepared foods. Cheese, for example, may contain up to a tablespoon of salt per pound. In some of Hans Selye's stress-theory experiments, he demonstrated that many heart attacks are caused by a sudden depletion of potassium in the cardiac muscle. Extreme stress can incite an oversecretion of ACTH in the pituitary. ACTH stimulates the adrenals to produce excessive amounts of corticosteroids, which, in turn, disturb the normal sodium-to-potassium ratio. Laboratory animals that were pretreated with potassium salts survived when exposed to stress levels that caused fatal coronary attacks in the controls.[333] The use of salt substitutes containing potassium chloride is a simple way to offset our sodium burden. Some foods, especially bananas, are very rich in potassium.

We have already discussed the need for calcium in the maintenance of bones and cell membranes, and as an antistress agent. The average American diet provides less than 800 mg of calcium daily but our real needs appear to be between 1,000 and

2,000 mg. Typical American diets are rather high in phosphorus. Liver, lecithin, food yeasts, and wheat germ are especially rich in this mineral. The higher the phosphorus intake, the greater the calcium and magnesium requirements. If these are taken in abundance, extra calcium should be included. Adelle Davis recommends that a quarter cup of calcium lactate (or gluconate) and one tablespoonful of magnesium oxide be mixed with each pound of yeast or lecithin. These are sold at health-food stores. Magnesium, zinc, and vitamins C and D are needed for proper assimilation, distribution, and use of calcium. [71]

Magnesium works with calcium to reduce stress. It also helps keep cholesterol levels down. We need about 50 mg of magnesium for every 100 mg of calcium taken. [78] Magnesium gluconate or lactate can be obtained inexpensively at health-food stores. Magnesium oxide is also available, but it tends to neutralize stomach acids unless hydrochloric-acid tablets are taken with it. [72] It may also have a laxative effect.

Zinc is proving to be important in the control of aging and age-related diseases. It is involved in DNA and RNA activities, is essential for protein synthesis, and promotes rapid healing of broken bones, burns, cuts, and bruises. It benefits the immune system, helps break down fats, and lowers cholesterol. There is growing evidence that it can assist in preventing age-induced prostatitis and rheumatoid arthritis. There is a competitive relationship between zinc and copper in the tissues. Although copper is an essential mineral, we usually get more than enough in our diets, and sometimes dangerous amounts from tap water. Excessive copper in the tissues can lead to hardening of the arteries, high blood pressure, kidney disease, psychoses, early senility, and other disorders of aging. [153, 267, 273, 280] It acts as a catalyst to cause rapid peroxidation of lipids, and increases the proliferation of free radicals. Superfluous copper is stored mostly in the liver and the brain. Schizophrenics have higher than normal amounts of copper in the brain. [280] Statistically, they also have shorter lifespans than normal people. Hoffer and Osmond suggest that this may be due to increased free-radical production. [154] Excessive copper in the liver inhibits the formation of an enzyme that breaks down serotonin, the neurohormone that has been blamed for activating the aging signal in the hypothalamus. Zinc, on the other hand, is needed in the structure of this enzyme. The average need for copper is about 2 mg a day. The average intake is between 3 and 5 mg. [274] The normal zinc-to-copper ratio in humans is 14 to 1; [281] so we need 40 to 70 mg of zinc each day to balance our copper intake. Manganese helps zinc to lower copper levels. It is also involved in acetylcholine storage and in enzymes that control the oxidative processes of the cell. We need at least 4 mg of this mineral each day, but the optimal dosage is believed to be around 15 to 25 mg. [283]

"I am particularly concerned about the need for better practical nutrition education for our doctors. The advice of family doctors carries a great deal of weight with most people. But, unfortunately, many doctors simply do not receive sufficient training in nutrition while they are at medical school to enable them to give the sound advice on nutrition that we urgently need."

Senator Richard S. Schweiker, *Prevention* (Oct. 1972)

Unless chromium is well-supplied in the diet, it decreases in the cells with age.[206] It is also needed for protein synthesis, and helps reduce cholesterol and prevent hardening of the arteries. The recently discovered glucose-tolerance factor (GTF) contains chromium. This vitamin-like substance enhances the efficiency of insulin, and can prevent diabetes and hypoglycemia. GTF is found in brewer's yeast. Absorption is fairly good (10 to 25 per cent). Intestinal bacteria can synthesize GTF from chromium salts, niacin, and amino acids, but uptake of these salts is poor (1 to 3 per cent).[287] If the diet is wholesome and includes at least two tablespoonfuls of brewer's yeast daily, chromium needs are likely to be filled. If yeast is not used, 250 to 1,000 mcg of chelated chromium can be supplemented. Prolonged use of more than 5 mg (5,000 mcg) can produce toxic side effects.

Most people know how important iron is in carrying oxygen in the blood, but few understand how to obtain it dietetically. There is no shortage of iron in most food, and supplements are rarely needed. Deficiencies of iron are most often due to the difficulty with which it is assimilated. Acidic foods, such as sour fruits, yogurt, kefir, and buttermilk, assist absorption, whereas sweets with meals inhibit it. Ascorbic acid increases iron absorption so much that nonanemic persons on megadosages of vitamin C should be cautious about taking iron supplements. *Too much iron can be toxic*. The recommended daily allowance is 10 to 18 mg. If all other nutritional factors are in order, this is usually quite enough. Since most iron-deficiency symptoms are caused by poor use of the mineral rather than by an insufficiency, they can be rectified with an all-round good diet that includes plenty of vitamins C, B6, and E.[73, 284] If iron supplements are taken, they should be in a chelated form, such as ferrous peptonate. Ferrous sulfate should never be used, since it destroys vitamin E and can be fatal in dosages exceeding 900 mg.[161, 169, 392] Unfortunately, many popular supplemental formulas, such as Geritol, contain as much as 50 mg of the sulfate per tablet.

Cobalt has already been discussed in connection with vitamin B12. Only small amounts (8 to 10 mcg) of this element are required. Excesses can be toxic. If the diet is wholesome, especially if brewer's yeast is taken, there is usually no need for supplements.

Iodine deficiency can result in hypothyroidism, the symptoms of which mimic aging. About 150 mcg of supplemental iodine will rectify the deficiency, but larger amounts will not slow the normal aging process.

Molybdenum has been overlooked as a micronutrient until recently. It appears to play a fundamental role in controlling aging. It is a part of xanthine oxidase and other enzymes. Tungsten can replace molybdenum in these enzymes and disrupt their functions; this would ultimately result in abnormal copper accumulations and more rapid peroxidation of lipids. It is difficult to know if you are getting too much tungsten, but if you are getting plenty of molybdenum, the tungsten should present no problem. Molybdenum is a powerful agent for reducing copper levels. Large amounts of it given to black sheep will cause such a copper depletion that their wool becomes white. By alternately decreasing and increasing copper levels, one can produce black-and-white-banded wool. Molybdenum also protects against cancer of the stomach and esophagus, helps keep amounts of uric acid down, decreases the incidence of dental caries, and increases muscle tone. A deficiency can cause poor sexual functioning in older men. The minimum daily need appears to be about 120 mcg, and 15 mg have been given therapeutically. A daily dosage of 500 to 1,000 mcg can be used as a supplement. [177, 285]

Vanadium is another micronutrient that has recently gained recognition. It inhibits cholesterol production and helps to prevent gallstones. The daily requirement is not yet known, but since it has practically no toxicity, 500 to 1,000 mcg can be taken. [160, 286]

Other minerals that are needed in human nutrition include tin, nickel, and arsenic. Little is known about our requirements for these, but only traces are needed, and we doubtlessly already get enough.

Aluminum, cadmium, lead, mercury, bismuth, and other nonnutritional metallic elements occur as contaminants in our food, water, and air. Some of these appear to have nutritional functions in very minute quantities, but our intake usually exceeds the required amounts and often reaches toxic levels. These elements accumulate in the tissues, hasten aging, and shorten lifespan. [329] They also interfere with brain functioning and may often be a cause of premature mental senility. Vitamin C assists in their removal. Other minerals which compete with them for sites in the body can be very effective in getting rid of them. Calcium, for instance, displaces lead; and zinc displaces cadmium. [51, 207] Selenium combines with methyl mercury, rendering it soluble for excretion. [207] Aluminum cooking utensils, buffered aspirins, antacids, and baking powders that contain aluminum hydroxide should not be used. The use of bismuth salts for periods of about a month can be helpful in healing gastric ulcers, but prolonged use can result in bismuth poisoning. The indiscriminate use of bismuth products, such as Pepto-Bismol, can be dangerous in this respect. Zinc, calcium, and magnesium, in combination, help the body to get rid of bismuth. [288]

---

As has rightly been said, it is better to eat junk foods and get adequate exercise, than to eat health foods and get no exercise at all. Aside from its many well-known benefits, exercise helps bring nutritional components to all the tissues and enables the tissues to make

*continued*

full use of them. It also helps remove toxic wastes from the body. In a sense, exercise may be regarded as a component of nutrition; but like food, it is something to be taken in satisfying amounts, and not overindulged in.

Although science has uncovered volumes of information on nutrition, there is still much to be learned. It is probable that not all the vitamins and other essential components have yet been discovered. It can be reasonably assumed, though, that they occur in many of our foods. A varied diet is generally recommended to ensure substantial amounts of both known and unknown materials. To be certain that adequate quantities of the known vitamins and minerals are received, supplements can be taken, as suggested here. However, until science has learned all there is to know about our nutritional needs, it should not be assumed that these supplements can entirely replace the vitamins, minerals, and other components that we derive from nature.

# Chapter Seven

# Is Aging a Disease?

## Autoimmune Theories of Aging and Slow Viruses

*So far, we have examined a few ways that we can slow down some aspects of aging and alleviate several age-related problems. But even if we could stop all unwanted oxidation and free-radical reactions in the body and rectify all cross-links, we would still grow old and die. The process would take a little longer, and we might be spared many of the discomforts of aging. We could probably retain good health, vigor, and a fairly youthful appearance for over a century. But the Grim Reaper would still have many weapons against which we'd remain defenseless.*

*Death, however, is not something apart from ourselves, a foreign invader from a distant shore. He is as much a part of us as life. Many of the very things that give us life and protect us from losing it also, in time, bring us death.*

*The immune system is the weapon that nature has given us to defend ourselves against toxins and diseases. Eventually, though, it turns on us and destroys us. The sword of life becomes the sword of death.*

*Science has begun to make some headway in learning to prevent unwanted changes in the defense system. We may never find a way to entirely prevent its decline, but we may soon have some ways to delay the event. And that is worth looking forward to.*

The body's immunological defense system is like a police force or militia. It is equipped and programmed to detect and destroy both foreign invaders and internal criminal upstarts. The invaders may be harmful bacteria, fungi, or viruses; the internal criminals, tumors or newly formed cancers. Like most powers entrusted with such responsibilities, it usually works for the general benefit of the organism which houses it. Were it absent, the body would be hopelessly vulnerable to attack from both without and within. But also like some police and military forces, it can get out of hand

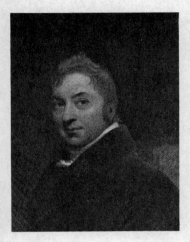

*Edward Jenner*

and turn against the entity it was created to protect. This reversal appears to be one of the ruinous events that contribute to aging.

Because the body's immune system is not concretely visible to the unaided eye, physicians of the past were not fully aware of its existence. Nevertheless, they were aware of some of its manifestations. Early records show that doctors have known for many centuries that persons who had recovered from a plague were protected from a second attack. During the late eighteenth century, some physicians began to gear their thinking in terms of this phenomenon, and attempted to understand its workings and find ways to apply its principles to saving lives.

One English physician named Edward Jenner had observed that smallpox was rare among milkmaids. Harmless cowpox sores on the hands of these ladies were a common occurrence, however. Jenner surmised that something in cowpox was protecting them against the more virulent disease. In 1796, he infected an eight-year-old boy with cowpox, and found that this made the child resistant to smallpox. This was the first man-made vaccine. *

Since Jenner's discovery, scientists have conquered many other disease viruses by developing vaccines against them, either from a weaker strain of the virus, or from dead or nearly dead viruses. The principle, however, was always the same: when the body is infected with a harmless form of a virus, the immunologic defense systems develop antibodies to protect against deadly forms. The technique led to the conquest of diphtheria by Von Behring in 1901, and of polio by Jonas Salk in the 1950s. It is now showing promise in coping with some cancer-causing viruses.

Essentially, the immune system is a biological protective organization to distinguish self from nonself. When it is functioning properly, it does no harm to the body's native protein. But it will recognize, attack, and destroy foreign proteins, like those in newly formed cancer cells or trespassing bacteria and viruses. It may also attack other large, foreign molecules, including certain polysaccharides and nucleic acids. This talent for detection and deletion usually serves to protect the host organism and maintain its structural integrity. Sometimes, though, it can work against the host. The well-known problem of organ-transplant rejection is entirely immunological. Unless the donor has the same genetic makeup as the recipient, as in an identical twin or possibly a close relative, the transplant is likely to be rejected. To prevent this, the patient is usually given drugs that suppress the immune defenses. Unfortunately, this leaves the system vulnerable to invasion by disease-causing microorganisms. Similarly, there are many dis-

---

* For many centuries before this, Oriental physicians had had some success immunizing patients against smallpox by using infectious material from milder cases of the disease. Sometimes it worked; sometimes it killed. These doctors never found ways to improve their technique, and there was no further progress in the ancient Asian art of vaccination.

eases, such as rheumatoid arthritis, rheumatic heart disease, multiple sclerosis, SLE (systemic lupus erythmatosus), glomerulonephritis, and some types of anemia, in which the immune system fails to recognize its own protein structures and attacks them. These are called autoimmune diseases.

One of the main figures in the immune system is a type of white blood cell known as the lymphocyte. There are about one trillion lymphocytes in the human body at any single time, circulating in the bloodstream or residing in the lymphoid tissues. Approximately ten million of them die and are replaced every minute. They are formed in the bone marrow as immature stem cells. Some of them mature in the bloodstream and become B-cells. Others pass through the thymus gland in the upper chest cavity and mature into T-cells.

When a foreign substance, or antigen, appears in the body, a biochemical alarm is given. One of the first duties of the T-cell is to act as a sentry and detect the antigen's presence. The T-cells then produce mediators, which summon B-cells, histiocytes, macrophages, and other warrior cells to the site of infection, and increase their activity and aggressiveness. The T-cells not only act as sentries and directors, but also manufacture chemical agents that destroy invading bacteria and fungi.

Plasma cells, which are derived from B-cells, produce antibodies. These are globular proteins called immunoglobulins, found in the gamma globulin fraction of the blood. Plasma cells produce only one type of antibody per cell, but the number of different antibodies possible is very large. When an antigen appears in the system, the cell that produces the particular antibody against that antigen is stimulated to divide and produce a clone of cells, which makes large amounts of that antibody. This selective propensity for producing particular antibodies is sometimes called an "immunologic memory." It is this phenomenon that makes vaccination and acquired immunity possible.

There is a lock-and-key relationship between antigen and antibody. A specific antibody shape exists to fit each antigen shape. When an antigen is encountered, the matching antibody connects with it and destroys it. This usually works for the well-being of the host, but sometimes not. Two familiar situations in which the immune system distresses the body are allergy and anaphylaxis. Allergy is a mild overreaction to a foreign substance that occurs when three-way links are formed between antigens, antibodies, and the mast cells, resulting in an excessive release of histamines and other chemical weapons. Anaphylaxis is a similar response, but is more severe and often results in death. It is a curiosity of semantics that when a reaction of the body's defenses is desirable, we call it immunity; when it is undesirable, we call it sensitivity. Yet they are biologically the same event.

During adolescence, the efficiency of the immune system is at its peak. After that there is a gradual decline. As the organism

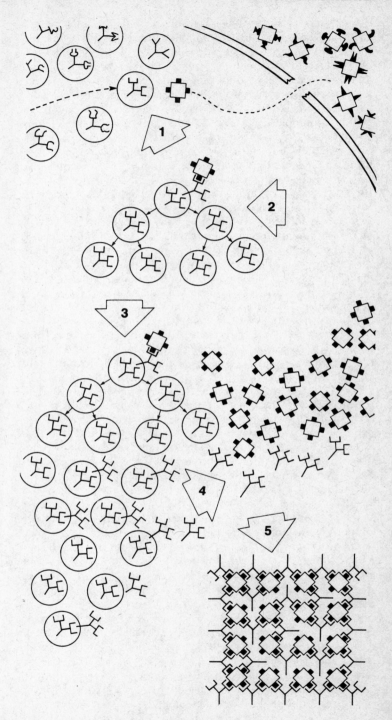

*Immunologic memory.*

(1) An antigen is recognized as a foreign material by a cell which already has a matching "lock" to the antigen "key."

(2) This cell is stimulated to divide and produce a clone of that cell.

(3) Years later, if one of these selected cells encounters the same antigen, the cell reacts to the antigen, and cell division is stimulated.

(4) This produces an increase in the population of that cell, and enough antibodies can be produced to cope with larger amounts of the antigen. These antibodies are proteins which can circulate in the bloodstream and can act at a place far from the cells that produced them.

(5) If the antigen has two or more sites at which the antibody can bind, a large network will form, immobilizing the antigen until the body removes the mass.

ages, the system is less able to cope with foreign invaders. What is worse, the immune cells and antibodies lose their ability to distinguish foreign cells and antigens from the body's own cells, proteins, and other materials. The defense system then begins to turn against the organism it was designed to protect. Because of this failure, autoimmune diseases are most common in the later years of life.

Around the same time, other age-related changes can intensify the problems caused by these autoimmune disorders. Free-radical damage to the tissues and the DNA results in improperly constructed proteins, which are truly foreign to the immune system. The system usually attacks and destroys them, and thus maintains the structural integrity of the tissues by removing flawed materials. But if this reaction is carried too far, it can overwhelm the entire organism.

The weakening of the senile immune system is largely due to a failure in T-cell function. The thymus gland begins to shrink early in life. It is the hormone thymosin from this gland that causes the stem cells from the bone marrow to mature into T-cells. As the body ages, less thymosin can be produced by this shrinking gland, and T-cell efficiency falls. Furthermore, changes in the aging pituitary gland cause the release of a blocking factor that inhibits the formation of thymosin. The resultant T-cell deficiency not only weakens the body's defenses, but also contributes to the upswing of autoimmune disorders. Some types of T-cells, known as suppressor lymphocytes, prevent overproduction of antibodies by the plasma cells. When antibody formation is not properly monitored and controlled, the probability of autoimmune diseases increases. The thymosin-blocking factor may be one of the hypothesized "death hormones" that many investigators have been trying to discover.

Several things can be done to hinder the weakening of the immune system and prevent it from becoming the body's ultimate enemy. Removal of the pituitary has resulted in some rejuvenation of the immune system in experimental animals. The operation has also been performed on human subjects as a drastic clinical measure to stop the development of breast cancer and to prevent diabetes-induced blindness.[254] When the gland is removed, other essential pituitary hormones must be supplied by injection. Unfortunately, science has not yet discovered all the hormones secreted by this gland.

It was originally believed that stem cells had to pass through the thymus gland to mature into T-cells. It is now known that thymosin can mature them as they circulate in the bloodstream. A sharp decrease in blood levels of this hormone usually takes place between the ages of 25 and 45, and a gradual decline continues throughout the remaining years. When the hormone is given to cancer patients or to children with T-cell deficiencies, T-cell deficiency improves by as much as 500 per cent. It has no

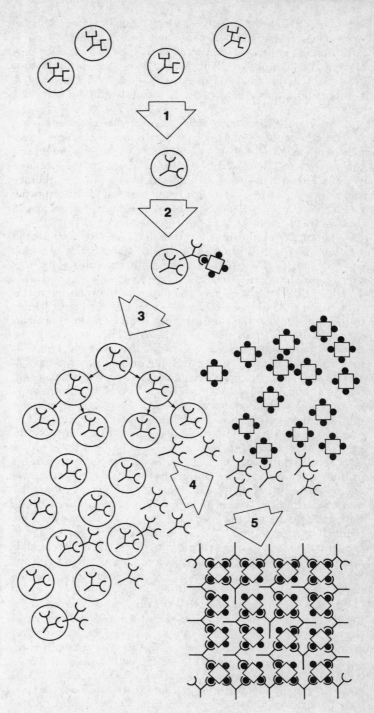

*Immune and autoimmune response.*
The antibody protein is actually "y"-shaped, with each of the two arms working as the "locks" for which the antigen carries the "key." The antigen molecule may also have more than one "key" area per molecule; so long chains and networks form when many "locks" are matched with many "keys."

(1) An autoimmune response can result if some change in the antibody-producing cell results in an antibody with an altered "lock."

(2) If this new "lock" fits a "key" which happens to be part of the normal body, (3) cell division is stimulated as if in response to a foreign antigen. The increased population of the cell then produces large amounts of the altered antibody, and (4) the antibody system is then attacking the "normal" molecules of its own body as if they were the original foreign antigen.

(5) As before, the attacked molecules may form a large network.

serious side effects, although a few patients have experienced mild localized skin reactions.

Thymosin was first isolated in 1965 by Allan L. Goldstein at Albert Einstein College of Medicine in New York. In 1977, the FDA gave Goldstein permission to conduct clinical trials with the hormone in the treatment of some autoimmune diseases. The Nutley, New Jersey, branch of Hoffman-LaRoche, Inc., is now producing large quantities of it.

Some initial experiments have been started to study thymosin's possibilities as an antiaging drug. Goldstein, now at the University of Texas Medical Branch in Galveston, and others have lengthened the lives of NZB mice with thymosin injections. [119, 120] This does not necessarily indicate that thymosin will extend the lives of other animals and human beings, however, since NZB mice have a hereditary susceptibility to autoimmune diseases, and do not ordinarily live out their potential lifespans. As a by-product of Goldstein's clinical trials, we may learn more about the relationships between thymosin, the immune system, and aging.

In another experiment, CBA/J mice were raised on a high-casein diet to induce amyloidosis. Injections of thymosin reduced the incidence and severity of amyloid formation in the animals. [119, 120, 176, 313, 325]

As was mentioned earlier, lymphocytes and their descendants are stimulated to develop almost exclusive "immunologic memories" against the antigens they encounter. The fact that lymphocytes also retain autoimmune "memories" makes them virtually useless in combatting invaders and turns them into dedicated enemies of the body. Several years ago, Takashi Makinodan at NIH infected young mice with a specific strain of bacteria, allowed them to develop immunity to it, and injected old mice with their lymphocytes. When he infected the old mice with lethal doses of the bacteria, they resisted the disease. More recently, Makinodan took lymphocytes from young animals and stored them in deep freeze at −196°C. When the animals were older and their defense systems were failing, he thawed the cells and reinjected them. Their immune systems were rejuvenated. He suggests that after further study, humans may be able to store their young lymphocytes in a cell bank and draw upon them as needed in old age. These lymphocytes would be free of defects and autoimmune memories. [394]

Makinodan has also revitalized the immune system by giving animals dosages of the antioxidant 2-MEA (2-mercaptoethylamine). [394] When selenium and vitamin E are taken together, they can stimulate the production of antibodies. [17] Vitamin E, selenium, and 2-MEA may be of some benefit to longevists who are trying to maintain a youthful immune system. If the current theories about thymosin inhibitors as a type of "death hormone" are correct, there may be several other things that can be done to prevent the decline of the immune system. These possibilities are explored in the next several chapters. [187, 326, 394]

## Slow Viruses

It has been speculated that slow-acting viruses may involve the immune system in more autodestructive episodes than we have already considered. An acute virus infection usually kills the infected cell within 10 to 48 hours, because the virus takes control of the cell's machinery and uses it to produce proteins and other components for virus replication. When the new viruses are produced, the cell breaks open, releases them, and perishes.

Slow viruses also alter the host cell's genes, but do not inhibit its synthesis of RNA. They continue to live in the cell for many years without killing it, and almost always alter the protein composition of the cell's outer membrane surface. This renders the cell and its progeny subject to attack by the immune system. Sometimes, even though the virus infection itself is fairly harmless, the immune system will destroy the infected cells. Occasionally, side reactions from the immune system's responses will result in life-threatening complications. The antibodies that are produced to combat lymphocytic choriomeningitis (LCM) combine with the virus to form virus-antibody complexes. These unusual structures become trapped in the capillaries of the kidneys and cause an inflammatory kidney disease called glomerulonephritis.

Some viruses depress the ability of the immune system to produce antibodies against other viruses. A slow-acting but persistent virus may cause sustained aberrations in the immune system that can result in multiple complications. Researchers now believe that many of the autoimmune diseases associated with aging are side reactions to viruses. Some investigators are beginning to suspect that the aging process itself—or at least some aspects of it—can be attributed to the immune system's responses to certain slow viruses. More findings in this line of research are anticipated during the next few years. [158]

# Chapter Eight

# "Death Hormones" and Aging Clocks

*Hormones stimulate the various processes of life, awaken them from dormancy, and set them in motion. If aging isn't a disease but merely a stage in the cycle of life, why shouldn't hormonal substances be involved?*

*Declining hormone production and failure to make full use of hormones are known to occur with age. There now appear to be hormone-like substances that signal many of the body's factories to shut down and aging changes to take place. The degrees to which these so-called "death hormones" contribute to aging cannot be fully known until we have learned to control them. In fact, we can control them now to some extent, and should be able to control them completely in the near future.*

*The trouble seems to start in the hypothalamus, the mysterious regulatory organ in the brain that we encounter often in this book. Other organs play secondary roles, and some aspects of aging may begin in the individual cells of the body. One of gerontology's big questions is whether the central control in the brain or the cellular level of control is more to blame for aging.*

*In this chapter we will consider arguments that attempt to pinpoint the location of the aging clock, along with several strategies that may be able to delay its effects. Most of the arguments and strategies touch on the concept that aging may be caused by hormones or hormone-like substances that the body generates during the later stages of life.*

## Obsolescence

One thing the American automotive industry has done for human consciousness is to give us a thorough and realistic understanding of the concept of built-in obsolescence. Wherever it is desired to continuously replace the old with the new, the specifications of

"Lifespan is not the preferred unit of measure. . . . The number of years we live is not too important if they are miserable years; our goal is to live better longer."

Richard A. Passwater,
*Supernutrition*

each unit, be it an automobile, an animal, or a human being, must include some means of assuring its timely dissolution after a reasonable period of use. Although most of us realize that our motor vehicles could be better built for longer wear, we have come to accept in our four-wheeled friends what we have always taken for granted in our transient selves: limited durability; guaranteed impermanence.

Compared to the human body, the automobile is a simple device. Old parts can be readily replaced, and the machine can be maintained for years in close to mint condition. The owner can do much to delay the date of his vehicle's demise, but—without ultimately replacing each and every part—the subtle destructiveness of time will eventually do its job. The human body may also be protected against early ruin if its owner takes care of it and includes the proper amounts of supplements, meganutrients, antioxidants, and free-radical deactivators in his diet. These and similar measures should add a few decades to the average life expectancy, prevent premature decline, and improve the health and vitality of life's later years. But only a little time is gained. Nothing is achieved that hasn't happened before. People have lived to be vigorous centenarians without following any special life-extension programs. There are, in fact, many indications that under ideal conditions the normal human lifespan should be 100 to 120 years, with reasonably decent health prevailing until close to the end.

The various animal studies that we have discussed so far strongly suggest that we can attain centenarian longevity by proper care of the body and the use of dietary antioxidants. But there is no reason to expect that any such measures can extend our lives much beyond this maximum. No matter what we do to prevent lipid peroxidation, environmental poisoning, nutritional deficiency, degenerative diseases, and immune-system failures, our lifespans are limited by other, more subtle factors. Somewhere in the body there seems to be a self-destruct mechanism that is set, like a time bomb, to go off after a given number of years, if something else has not already done the job. Detecting and disarming this biological time bomb is the primary concern of gerontologists working with the so-called aging-clock hypothesis. Those who are wagering their time and energy on this hypothesis offer many different speculations about the location and nature of this autodestruct mechanism. Some believe that it operates through the endocrines, activated by a signal from a control center in the brain. Others think that each cell is programmed to die, or to bring about the death of the whole organism at an approximately appointed time. Even within each of these camps, there is no general agreement about the brain, endocrine, or cellular sites.

## The Central Aging-Clock Hypothesis

Among those who adhere to the central aging-clock hypothesis, Caleb Finch of USC blames the thyroid gland. Hypothyroidism (insufficient thyroxin production) causes symptoms like those of aging, such as wrinkled skin, gray hair, senile dementia, and poor resistance to disease and stress. When thyroxin injections are given, these symptoms disappear, and the patient assumes a more youthful state, appropriate to his actual age. Near the turn of the last century, this phenomenon led some scientists to believe that they might similarly rejuvenate an aging person with this treatment. All experiments failed, however, and often did more harm than good. The problem in aging is not that thyroxin production dwindles, but that the tissues lose their ability to take up the hormone from the bloodstream and make use of it. [94]

W. Donner Denckla of the La Roche Institute of Molecular Biology believes that the difficulty may be due to the secretion of a pituitary hormone which does not inhibit thyroid secretions, but acts on the cell membrane to prevent the assimilation of thyroxin into the cell. He calls this blocking hormone DECO, which is an acronym for "decreasing consumption of oxygen."[80] Some gerontologists (not Denckla) call this and other possible blocking factors "death hormones." We use this term cautiously and in quotation marks throughout this book when speaking of any specific (or unspecific) pituitary substances that contribute to the decline of life.

In 1975, Denckla rejuvenated the cardiovascular and immunological systems of aging rats by removing their pituitaries and administering thyroxin. When he gave the thyroid hormone to rats whose pituitaries were intact, no such revitalization took place.[81] This is a harsh approach to rejuvenation, particularly when the pituitary is not the real culprit.

Although the pituitary is the master gland that directs the activities of the endocrine system, it is controlled by the hypothalamus. Substances known as releasing factors trickle down from the hypothalamus to the nearby pituitary and activate the release of one or several of its hormones, which, in turn, stimulate or inhibit the production of hormones in other glands; or prevent them from affecting the cells or organs that they would normally act upon.

The hypothalamus is the body's organ of homeostasis. It maintains the equilibrium of most biological processes. Its secretions keep internal temperature, blood pressure, thirst, hunger, sexual appetites, chemical and water balances, menstrual cycles, sleeping and waking patterns, and numerous other activities functioning normally. For the hypothalamus to do this, it must be sensitive to biochemical changes that signify slight deviations in these functions. Too much or too little of a particular hormone in

"There is no theoretical reason why in the next century we shouldn't live to the age of 150 or beyond."

W. Donner Denckla, quoted in *The Detroit News* (April 1, 1979)

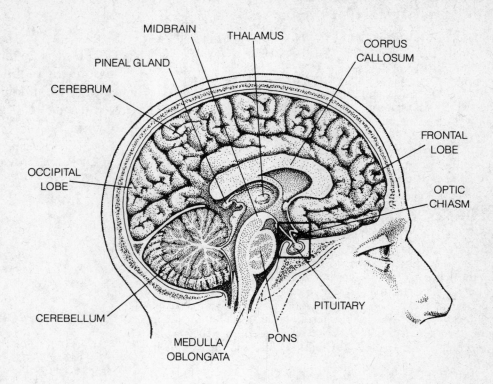

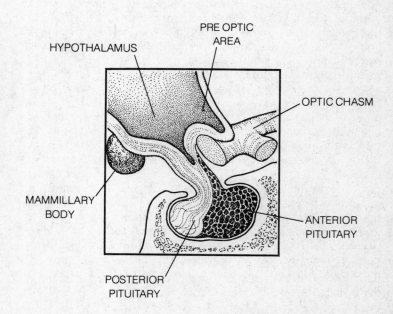

*Brain and pituitary.*

The hypothalamus plays a primary role in converting information from the brain into hormonal body responses. Releasing factors (small protein-like molecules) from the hypothalamus initiate hormonal changes in the pituitary (considered the master gland). The releasing factors themselves are regulated by complex interactions from different parts of the brain; so the master gland is actually under control of the brain via the hypothalamus. The anatomical relation of the brain, hypothalamus, and pituitary is shown here.

the tissues influences the hypothalamus to secrete more or less of specific releasing factors and inhibiting factors which bring about the adjustment. This control and feedback system suggests several approaches for gerontologists who are trying to cope with hormones that may cause aging. They might isolate DECO and other "death hormones," and find substances that can break them down; they might isolate the pertinent releasing and inhibiting factors, and learn to neutralize them; or they might determine what conditions in the hypothalamus make it secrete these factors, and discover ways to avoid such conditions.

Pituitary hormones and the enzymes that negate them are complex substances, difficult to isolate, and even more difficult to synthesize. Releasing and inhibiting factors are smaller, less complicated molecules.[124] These structures should be much easier to manufacture than the pituitary hormones themselves. Attempting to neutralize "death hormones" or their releasing factors might be an endless and self-defeating battle, however, since the hypothalamus, receiving no signal that it has produced enough of these factors, would continue relentlessly to manufacture them, perhaps at an increased rate. The most effective approach may be to control the conditions in the hypothalamus which influence secretion of the releasing factors. Several scientists, including Paola Timiras and Paul Segall of the University of California, Berkeley, have reasons to believe that one of these conditions is increasing levels of the neurohormone serotonin in the hypothalamic region. This and simultaneous decreases in dopamine were found to occur with age.[330, 331, 383] Stress, diet, atmospheric ionization, and a number of other factors appear to influence serotonin and dopamine levels. These matters are explored farther on in this chapter.

Another way to control the releasing factors might be to trick the hypothalamus into "thinking" that it has produced enough of them. If the structures of the "death hormones" can be determined, similar but slightly altered molecules could be synthesized. These misconstructed molecules would not be precise enough to do harm (block thyroxin uptake, etc.), but could be similar enough to mislead the hypothalamus with a chemical signal that it had secreted enough of the factors.

There are indications that aging may be brought on not only by increased production of "senile hormones," but also by reduced formation of "juvenile hormones." In a now famous experiment, Dietrich Bodenstein of the NIH Gerontology Research Center in Baltimore bored tiny holes in the backs of an old and a young cockroach, and joined their bloodstreams. The older insect gained an extended lifespan and recaptured many facets of youth, including the ability to regenerate severed limbs. This technique is known as parabiosis.[27] Frederic C. Ludwig of the University of California, Irvine, has succeeded in rejuvenating parabiotic rats and extending their lifespans.[191, 215, 314] It is amazing that these experiments were so successful, when the animals were under the constant stress of being interconnected. If the same thing could be done without the burden of being man-made Siamese twins, the results might be even better. This could be accomplished in humans by giving periodic transfusions of young blood to older persons, or by isolating and synthesizing the youth factors for injection.

Remarkable results have been obtained with another technique, called plasmapheresis, which means withdrawal of blood. Two pints of blood at a time are withdrawn from the body. The red blood cells are separated from the plasma under refrigeration in a centrifuge. They are then returned to the body in two pints of a physiologically neutral solution. The new plasma that the body is forced to produce has many youthful characteristics. Also, the rate of cell growth and division is speeded up throughout the body, cholesterol levels are lowered, and cholesterol metabolism is altered to resemble that of a younger person. Volunteers for plasmapheresis experiments also look and feel better after the treatment. This procedure removes toxins and old, defective soluble proteins. If "death hormones" do exist, they too may be removed. In lieu of plasmapheresis facilities, a person could donate blood to a blood bank once a month. Four donations of a pint each should achieve plasmapheresis of 50 per cent of the total blood volume. Norman Orentreich, a leader in this field, says that if fifty million dollars were spent on plasmapheresis research, we could double human lifespan by the year 2000. [192, 210]

Sir Macfarlane Burnet, one of Australia's top gerontologists, * and several other workers who are pursuing the central aging-clock hypothesis believe that the thymus is the cause of aging. [312] The fact that this organ shrinks as the body matures lends some support to their belief. Since the thymus and its hormone thymosin are responsible for the functioning of the immunological system, and since failures in this system are at least a part of the aging problem, their suspicions cannot be entirely discounted. The experiments of Allan L. Goldstein, mentioned in Chapter 7, may soon shed some light on the significance of thymosin as an anti-aging drug, but immunological failure does not currently appear to be the key cause of aging. Thymosin may help the system defend itself against cancer and other diseases that attack the aged, and thymus failure may contribute to aging, but we don't know what causes the organ's shrinking and decreased output. Experimental evidence suggests that these changes are induced by pituitary secretions that are activated by hypothalamic releasing factors.

---

* He was also the first to propose the now-accepted selective theory of immunology.

# The Cellular Aging-Clock Hypothesis

Those who regard the individual cells as the site of the biological aging clock frequently cite the Hayflick Limit as confirmation for their view. The maximum of about fifty doublings in cultured embryonic human fibroblasts seems to indicate that cells age independently. Since there are no endocrines to produce "death hormones" in a tissue culture, the mechanism for scheduled obsolescence, they say, must reside in the cells themselves.

There are a number of findings, however, that weaken Hayflick's conclusions and cast doubt on the cellular aging-clock hypothesis. The methods used to keep the Hayflick cultures alive are thought to be faulty. Lowering the oxygen content of the medium or adding antioxidants has greatly extended the number of cell divisions. [252, 253] The fact that muscle cells, which are not inclined to divide in the adult body, do so *in vitro*, along with the discovery that uncontaminated chick-embryo extracts — despite the invalidation of Carrel's experiments — do increase tissue-culture lifespans, [9] has further contradicted both the Hayflick Limit and the concept of a cellular aging mechanism.

Several other studies also tend to bolster the central-clock hypothesis and deflate the cellular one. In 1966, at the University of Milan, the team of Pecile, Müller, and Falconi transferred the pituitary of an old female rat to the body of a young one, and caused the latter's ovaries to atrophy. [264] During the same year, in England, Talbert and Krohn transplanted nonreproductive ova from an aging female rat to the ovaries of a young one. After fertilization, a healthy litter was born. [379] In 1973, Tauchi and Hasegawa found that while the liver cells of the older of a para- biotic pair of rats develop more youthful characteristics, the younger one's liver cells show signs of rapid aging. [380]

The publication of the commitment theory, in late 1977, seemed to deal the final blow to Hayflick's concepts and the cell-clock hypothesis. According to its authors, Robin Holliday and G.M. Tarrant, a newly started tissue culture contains cells that are committed to decline and perish after a given number of divisions, and others that are uncommitted and potentially immortal. During cell division, more committed cells are formed, and all replications of these are also committed. The behavior of a cell culture greatly depends on the proportion of committed to uncommitted cells. As the cells proliferate, the population of committed cells increases, while that of the uncommitted cells diminishes. The standard practice of periodi- cally pruning cultures further reduces the original number of uncommitted cells. The theory is well-supported by experimental findings. [159]

More recently, workers at MIT who have been experiment- ing with transplanted fibroblast colonies have demonstrated that this process of subculturing may induce further division. They suspect that the termination of proliferation is a stage in cell differentiation rather than a result of senescence. [11]

Most evidence, at this time, suggests that aging is largely effected by the hypothalamus and pituitary, rather than by a mechanism within the individual cells of the body. Leonard Hayflick's studies have been the major premise for the cellular aging hypothesis. Although some of his theories are beginning to crumble, gerontologists cannot entirely dismiss the idea that the cell may hold the secret of aging. The cells are the life of the body. Much of the aging process has to occur within them. The question is how much of the aging phenomenon is initiated through the cells, and exactly where, how, and why does this take place?

Denham Harman suspects that the mitochondria are where aging begins. Within these elongated organelles, 90 per cent of the body's oxidative processes are conducted. Harman believes that this much oxidation would greatly increase free-radical pro- liferation in the mitochondria, and disrupt their function as energy transformers. [137] Dorothy Travis of the Gerontology Research Center thinks that aging may be due to an interaction between the lysosomes and the mitochondria. While studying the heart cells of aging rodents, she observed rows of lysosomes attached to the mitochondria. It is known that lysosome activity increases during the second half of an animal's life. Perhaps both Harman and Travis are correct. Free-radical damage to the mem- branes of both organelles may induce the lysosomes to cling to the mitochondria, and these scavenger units may then do further damage.

Many believe that the DNA molecule itself carries the genetic program to destroy its creation at a more or less predeter- mined time. Since tendencies toward long or short lifespans are largely hereditary, this sounds reasonable. It is possible that intrinsically caused changes in the genes, or histone-induced changes in gene expression, directly effect aging. Or it may only be that from birth the genes dictate the nature and timing of the hypothalamic/pituitary aging clock and the other functionings within the body that interact with it. Whatever it is that makes us age, it is written in our genes, and it is here that we must finally seek the key to longevity. Perhaps by the time we find the genes that directly or indirectly cause the body to age, the new but growing science of genetic engineering will have found a way to control them.

## Mutual Effects

There is no reason why the two aging-clock hypotheses—or any other proposed causes of senescence—must be mutually exclu- sive. Nevertheless, even the best researchers tend to think in such terms, partly because the problem of controlling the aging process appears now to be so complex that gerontologists are trying to narrow it down to a few main causes. A logical approach to this is elimination of the less likely causes. From what we already know about biology, it is probable that both central and cellular aging clocks exist, and that aging is caused by a highly integrated series of interactions between these and other factors. Some longevists and gerontologists regard all the possible aging causes as a fail-safe system to guarantee built-in obsolescence. This is the same way that the automotive industry makes certain that old cars die off and are replaced by newer models. If one thing fails to go wrong with a motor vehicle, any number of things can be counted on to break down. Similarly, if a person isn't killed by accident or illness, free-radical damage may do the job soon enough. If this can be prevented, we can still expect the immune system to turn against the body. If this too is averted, "death hormones" from the hypothalamus and pituitary will probably finish us off. If even these can be controlled, the finite characteristics of the cells and the programming of the genes can be relied on to ensure that nature's plan for continuous turnover is not subverted.

"If life had been unnegated from the beginning, we should now be a solid ball of flesh expanding into the universe at a speed approximating that of light."

Dean Juniper,
*Man Against Mortality*

## Underfeeding

Curiously, the two most effective life-extension techniques — those which have doubled or tripled the normal lifespan — have been known for the longest time. Calorie restriction was discovered in the early 1930s and hypothermia (cooling the body temperature) in 1917. The only approaches that have surpassed these are variations, amplifications, or combinations of the two.

It is generally agreed that most Americans eat too much. Overeating and obesity tend to shorten life. Cutting down on excess calories and occasional fasting can help prevent premature death, but will not increase the average maximum lifespan.

Severe restriction of calories, protein, or certain amino acids can literally keep you a perennial child. But they are rough ordeals and may kill you first. Luckily, some alternative approaches are being found that should achieve the same results more safely and effectively.

During the late 1920s and early 1930s, Clive M. McCay at Cornell University observed that trout whose growth had been retarded by underfeeding lived longer than usual. Following this, he raised a group of newly weaned rats on a diet that was adequate in most respects, but contained only 30 per cent of the normal calorie requirement. Ordinarily, the mean lifespan of rats is about 600 days, and the average maximum lifespan is about 950 days. After 700 days McCay's rats not only were still alive, but had not even reached puberty. He then put them on a normal calorie diet.

They soon attained maturity, and from then on lived out typical adult lifespans. Most of the animals lived for a total of about 1,000 days, the longest lifespan being 1,465 days. This represents about a 66 per cent increase over the controls.[223]

More recently, Morris H. Ross of the Institute of Cancer Research in Philadelphia further amplified the caloric-restriction diet and achieved a 75 per cent increase in average lifespan. Some of his rats lived for more than 1,800 days, three times the mean lifespan of the controls.[314, 331] If human beings could do likewise, they might have lifespans of up to 180 years.

During the mid-1950s, Arthur V. Everitt studied the relationship between underfeeding and life extension. He and other investigators noticed many similarities in appearance between underfed rats and ones that had undergone hypophysectomy (surgical removal of the pituitary gland). It was also noted that underfeeding decreases production of some pituitary hormones. Everitt made a thorough study of the physiological effects of hypophysectomy on rats. He found that skeletal development and maturation are greatly slowed down, as is cross-linkage of collagen. Gradual senile kidney damage, common in aging rats, does not occur; nor is there the usual increase in heart size with age. The ability of the tissues to take up and utilize thyroxin does not decline as it would ordinarily. When the pituitaries of older rats were removed, their immune systems were often rejuvenated. Still, the hypophysectomized rats lived no longer than the controls. In fact, unless a small amount of corticosterone was added to their diet, they usually had shorter lifespans.[96, 249] Earlier we

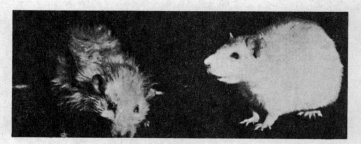

*Calorie restriction and longevity.*
McCay pioneered the research in life extension by calorie restriction in the 1930s. This photo shows the dramatic effect on the appearance and longevity of an animal raised on a diet restricted in calories but adequate in other nutrients.

The rats are the same age, 964 days old; the rat on the left, which was raised on a normal diet, died on the day the photo was taken. The rat on the right was raised on a calorie-restricted diet for 1,000 days, then put on a normal diet. It lived for nearly a year after this photograph was made.

mentioned similar experiments by Denckla in which hypophysectomy was combined with thyroxin injections. More recently,
Denckla, Parker, and others have been studying animals which
are given known pituitary hormones after hypophysectomy. [81, 254]

Various research workers have conducted experiments
restricting dietary components other than calories. In 1968,
D. S. Miller and P. R. Payne of Queen Elizabeth College in
London extended the lifespan of aging rats by 28 per cent after
putting them on a low-protein diet. [200] At the University of California in Berkeley, Paola Timiras and Paul Segall kept rats on an
otherwise adequate diet that contained only one sixth of the
normal requirement of the essential amino acid tryptophan.
Their results were comparable to McCay's. Tryptophan restriction was begun when the rats were three months old and was
continued for eleven months. Only one third of the animals
survived, but those that did had extended lifespans. One twenty-

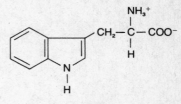

*Tryptophan*

Tryptophan is an essential amino
acid, which Paul Segall restricted
to low levels in his life-extension
experiments.

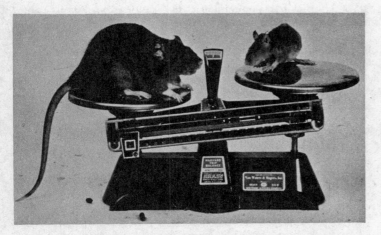

*Tryptophan restriction and
longevity.*

These two rats are the same age.
The rat on the left has been raised
on a normal diet; the rat on the
right was raised on a tryptophan-
deficient diet. Her development
has been slowed greatly, and she is
biologically still an adolescent.

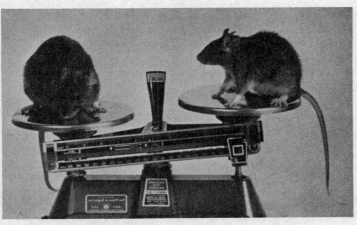

Now the rat on the right has been
switched over to the regular diet,
and has resumed normal development. But for her, the biological
clock had been halted. Whereas
normal rats stop bearing litters at
about 15 months of age, experimental animals like her have given
birth to litters at 28 months! In
human terms, this is roughly
equivalent to a 70-year-old woman
giving birth.

month-old female gave birth to a healthy litter, whereas normally rats have ceased to ovulate by the time they are seventeen months old. Near the end of their lives all the rats underwent accelerated decline. Throughout the experiment, they were undersized and scruffy looking, but after tryptophan levels were normalized, their appearance improved and they continued to grow toward the proper size. They were able to do this because rats, unlike many other animals, do not entirely cease growth after maturity. Mice do not resume growth upon restoration of adequate tryptophan; neither would humans.

As in McCay's experiments, the extension of lifespan was due primarily to delayed maturity, but Timiras and Segall believe that the results of their experiments were partly caused by the lowering of serotonin levels in the brain. High serotonin levels are believed to be one of the conditions that bring about the release of the so-called "death hormones." [330, 383]

At present, there is no safe way to apply the calorie- or tryptophan-restriction techniques toward the extension of human life. They would have to be started shortly after weaning and continued for thirty years or more. The mortality rate would be high, and if the person did survive, his mental, emotional, and social development would be distorted by the drastic experience. So would his physical development. Some minerals would be improperly distributed and deposited in the body, resulting in calcium loss in the bones and calcification of the arteries and kidneys. These problems could be rectified later with a corrective diet, but the individual's stature would still be permanently stunted.

The peoples of some areas of the world are reputed to be remarkably long-lived. Their longevity is often credited to their low caloric intake. It has been estimated that Hunza males consume a daily average of 1,900 calories; the people of the Caucasus, 1,700 to 1,900; and the villagers of Vilcabamba in the Andes of Ecuador, 1,200 to 1,700. In contrast, the average for American males of all ages is 3,300 a day. [332] This strongly suggests that the excessive eating habits of most Americans is not compatible with the goal of long life. The longevity of the Hunzas, Caucasians, and Vilcabambans, however, cannot be attributed to delayed maturity. Nor does the practice of occasional fasting for resting the digestive organs and helping the body to rid itself of toxic accumulations have anything in common with these long-term dietary-restriction experiments. Proper fasting methods are outlined in Chapter 11.

# Hypothermia

*Star Trek*'s Mr. Spock has given us the Vulcan salutation of greeting and farewell: "Live long and prosper." But one of our human salutations, "Be cool," may have already been saying the same thing, as well as offering a means of achieving it. Scientists now believe that if we could reduce our body temperature by just a few degrees, we would extend our lifespan to almost 300 years.

Hypothermia is an experimental life-extension technique that is often associated with calorie restriction. It involves the lowering of the internal body temperature by a few degrees. In 1917, Jacques Loeb and John H. Northrop at the Rockefeller Institute lengthened the lives of fruit flies by maintaining their environment at a temperature 6°C lower than normal, and shortened their lives by similarly raising the temperature.[213] Because fruit flies are cold-blooded organisms, their environmental temperature becomes their internal temperature.

Since 1917, other researchers have conducted similar experiments with other cold-blooded creatures and have achieved similar results. During the mid-1960s, Charles H. Barrows at Baltimore's Gerontology Research Center doubled the normal 18-day lifespan of tiny aquatic animals known as rotifers by lowering their water temperature 10°C. By simultaneously cutting their caloric intake in half, he was able to triple their lifespan.[10] Barnett Rosenberg and Gabor Kemeny at Michigan State University have achieved phenomenal life extensions using hypothermia on fruit flies. On the average, flies kept at 91°F body temperature lived 10 days; at 87.8°F, 20 days; at 80.6°F, 50 days; and at 77°F, 70 days.[174, 306] Dr. Rosenberg says that if all goes well with animal tests, drug-induced hypothermia could be tried on humans in about ten years. He believes that once this technique is perfected, it could extend human lifespan to about 200 years.

Walford and Liu doubled the lifespan of South American annual fish by cooling their water five degrees.[211, 212, 314] Walford finds that hypothermia, like caloric restriction, suppresses the immune system in a beneficial way. Animals that have been subjected to either of these techniques are less inclined to reject transplanted tissues, but, paradoxically, they are more resistant to tumors and infections. Unlike caloric restriction, hypothermia is most effective when applied during the second half of an animal's life, probably because autoimmune disorders increase at that time. Curiously, creatures that undergo hypothermia at middle age live longer than ones that are kept hypothermic from birth. Walford says that hypothermia is the greatest immunosuppressing measure known thus far. It is certainly the most effective life-extension technique known at this time. The normal human

"While it is doubtful that we can consider senescence and death as directly due to aging changes in the endocrine glands, such alterations may nevertheless play a very definite supporting role."

Thomas H. McGavack, Professor Emeritus of Clinical Medicine at New York Medical College body temperature of 37°C (98.6°F) allows a maximum lifespan of about 100 years. Walford estimates that a drop to 35°C would extend the maximum to 150 years; a drop to 33°C, to 180 years; and a drop to 31°C, to 270 years. He says that our normal body temperature is probably ideal for hunting and strenuous labor, and has been retained in our evolution as a prosurvival trait, but that it is not necessary or even desirable for twentieth-century man. [394]

These experiments have led some writers to suggest that living and sleeping in a cool environment can extend lifespan. If this were so, Eskimos would be long-lived, instead of short-lived. We are not cold-blooded. A person should live and sleep in a surrounding temperature that is comfortable. An extremely cool environment necessitates an increased metabolic rate and a high caloric intake, which can work against longevity. It also makes sleep uncomfortable and stressful.

The internal temperature of humans and other homeo-therms (warm-blooded organisms) does not depend on that of the environment, but is regulated by a thermostatic control center in the hypothalamus. To induce hypothermia in ourselves, we would have to manipulate this organ directly. Robert Meyers of Purdue has accomplished this with monkeys, and Rosenberg and Kemeny have done it with rats. [190, 314] Several drugs are known to lower the internal body temperature, including valium, barbiturates, chlorpromazine (Thorazine), marijuana derivatives, L-dopa, PCPA (parachlorophenylalanine), reserpine, disulfiram, methimazole (Tapazole), pimozide (a minor tranquilizer), neurotensin and bombesin (both naturally occurring peptides), and, to some extent, aspirin. Dr. Rosenberg has usually been cautious about discussing the drugs used in his hypothermia studies, probably more because of personal ethics than professional secrecy. No doubt, the good doctor does not want to encourage the abuse of such drugs among aspiring longevists. Neither do we. The correct dosage and usage of these substances for hypothermic life extension has not yet been established. There are also many uncertainties about the side effects of hypothermia in humans. Although short-term temperature reduction has been used for surgical and therapeutic purposes and has produced no lasting side effects, some gerontologists fear that prolonged hypothermia may result in hangover, sluggish behavior, and temporary IQ loss. Calorie restriction may cause body temperature to drop as much as three degrees, but this is often accompanied by unpleasant chills. It is possible, though, to prevent these with chlorpromazine (Thorazine), barbiturates, or other drugs. [199, 314]

There are several possible ways to lower human body temperature without use of drugs. It is likely that the hypothalamic thermostat could be controlled by biofeedback. Yogis can bring about drops of around a degree at will. [394] There is normally a fluctuation of about half a degree in humans, the highest temper-

"Man could add perhaps twenty-five years to his life if he could learn the hummingbird's trick and cool down at night."

Robert S. de Ropp,
*Man Against Aging*

atures being during the day and the lowest at night. There is also a parallel rise and fall of serotonin levels in the pineal gland.[401] Serotonin can cause a temperature increase of about a third of a degree.[150] Conversely, norepinephrine (noradrenaline) can decrease body temperature.[198]

Can the phenomenal life extensions from hypothermia be credited solely to its effect on the immune system? If they can, then the immune system must play a greater role in aging than we have previously ascribed to it. However, several other changes brought about by hypothermia could also explain its influence on longevity. For one thing, many aspects of metabolism are slowed down, but others are speeded up, in order (according to Denckla) to compensate for the loss of heat. Walford's annual fish had a higher ratio of soluble to insoluble (cross-linked) collagen than was typical for their age; this could signify a reduction of lipid peroxidation and free-radical reactions. The fact that Walford's fish also grew abnormally large may indicate a stimulation of the pituitary growth hormone, which some gerontologists believe to be a "youth factor." Hypothermic growth-hormone promotion and the relationship between serotonin and body temperature suggest that this technique may be another way of coping with "death hormones." *

Metabolic torpidation — somewhat related to hypothermia — includes hibernation (remaining in twilight sleep or torpor through the winter) and estivation (the same through the summer). These are natural habits of some animals. During hibernation, the aging rate may be reduced to as little as 5 per cent of normal. When animals are induced to hibernate for longer periods than usual, they tend to live longer. The substance that causes estivation to take place in the African lungfish has been isolated and injected into rats, effecting a 40 per cent reduction in their metabolic rate.[314, 377] Although it would be impractical and tedious for human beings to hibernate for long periods just to gain a few years of life, some of the principles involved could be used to improve the restorative qualities of sleep. This would increase health and might even lengthen life.

---

* Hypothermia has nothing in common with cryonics, the practice of deep-freezing a person immediately after death. The assumption of cryonics is that scientists and physicians in the future will be able to thaw and revive the frozen corpse and cure whatever caused its death. Several cryonics companies (see page 160 for names and addresses) are now freezing dead persons who have made the necessary previous arrangements.

## Air Ions and Serotonin

"Death is not absolute, but relative to the ability of existing technology to resuscitate."

Arthur Quaife,
ALCOR Conference

Electricity, like light, is all around us, even inside of us. All existence seems to be an electrical dance of positive and negative polarities. The Earth is electrically charged; so is the air we breathe. Weather changes often produce electrical changes. Our body chemistry involves interchanges of positive and negative charges, and the chemistry of the mind and body can be altered by changes in atmospheric electricity.

Negative-ion generators, which control this electricity, are now becoming popular. People who have installed these appliances in their homes, offices, and automobiles find that they feel less tense, more energetic, and generally healthier. Scientific studies support their observations. The ion-generator industry may soon enjoy a commercial boom comparable to that of waterbeds. There are also reasons to believe that these generators may slow down the aging process and extend lifespan.

Frequently, between spring and autumn, a strangely disturbing wind blows from the south across the dry lands of the Middle East, leaving physical, mental, and emotional havoc in its wake. In Israel it is known as the Sharav. In Arab countries it is called the Hamsin. Its deranging nature is like what some people experience when the moon is full, but more overwhelming. Even before the wind arrives, its effects can be felt. A few individuals, blessed with natural vitality, may find it stimulating and exhilarating. Others feel nothing at all unusual. But for many it is a sickening wind that drains them of their normal energies and makes them feel old before their time. Exhaustion, depression, insomnia, anxiety, irritability, and nausea are among the most common complaints when the Sharav is on its way. Many people experience breathing difficulties during this condition; those with asthma and other bronchial problems have some of their worst ordeals. Likewise, migraine sufferers are almost bound to feel its effects.

It has been noted that conflicts between Arabs and Jews in Jerusalem are more likely to occur during the advent of the Sharav. Suicides and acts of violence are also at their peak. the courts, long aware of this, tend to be lenient when trying crimes committed under its influence. Accidents, too, are more frequent during the Sharav, because it tends to fog alertness and slow down reaction time. Those who feel the effects of this wind are likely to be the same "weather-sensitive" people who feel the spell of the full moon, or become tense or depressed before an electrical storm.

The Arabs and the Jews are not the only peoples who are plagued by distressing winds. Another, known as the Föhn, blows through parts of Switzerland, Austria, and southern Germany. It brings weather-sensitive persons the same suffering that comes with the Sharav. Again, in these countries, the courts consider its influence when meting out justice. Many surgeons will not schedule serious operations during the Föhn. There is a tendency toward excessive bleeding at this time, and a patient's chance of survival is considerably lessened.[346]

Winds like these are often called Witches' Winds. They are known throughout the world. In southern France, there is the Mistral; in Italy, the Sirocco. Across the Rocky Mountains, during early spring, there is the Chinook; in southern California, the Santa Ana. It is almost always a warm, dry wind, frequently coming from the south or east, the notorious ill wind that blows no good.

In 1957, Dr. Felix G. Sulman, now head of the Department of Applied Pharmacology at the Hebrew University in Jerusalem, began his studies of the Sharav phenomenon. He had been researching the role of the neurohormone serotonin during pregnancy. Little was known about the functions of this substance at that time, and although they are better understood today, many questions remain. Serotonin is found in all tissues of the body except the amniotic fluid. The cells of the intestinal tract and the spleen are especially rich in it. It is a smooth-muscle and heart-muscle stimulant and a blood-vessel constrictor, is involved in the chemical transmission of nerve impulses, and is an essential brain amine and CNS (central nervous system) stimulant. When rats are rendered deficient in serotonin, they experience CNS depression. Clearly, serotonin is important in maintaining normal bodily functions, but excessive amounts of it can cause tension, raise blood pressure, increase sensitivity to pain, and inhibit healing of injuries. Usually MAO (monoamine oxidase) enzymes and other substances in the body will break down superfluous serotonin into harmless 5-HIAA (5-hydroxyindole acetic acid), which is excreted in the urine. Sulman tested two hundred Sharav victims and found that during the wind they produced an average of ten times the normal amount of serotonin, but their production of enzymes that can deactivate it to 5-HIAA only doubled at best.[57, 155, 184]

Later, Sulman became aware of the work of Albert P. Krueger, a brilliant microbiologist and experimental pathologist at the University of California, Berkeley. Krueger and his associate, Richard Smith, had been studying the effects of positive and negative ions on the biochemistry of mice. Ions are atoms whose normal electrical balance is upset because they have either lost or gained an electron, which has a negative charge. The air that we breathe is a mixture of several gaseous elements, mainly nitrogen and oxygen. Normally, each atom of any element contains a given number of positively charged protons within its

"There was a desert wind blowing that night. It was one of those hot dry Santa Anas that come down through the mountain passes and curl your hair and make your nerves jump and your skin itch. On nights like that every booze party ends in a fight. Meek little wives feel the edge of the carving knife and study their husbands' necks. Anything can happen."

Raymond Chandler,
*Red Wind*

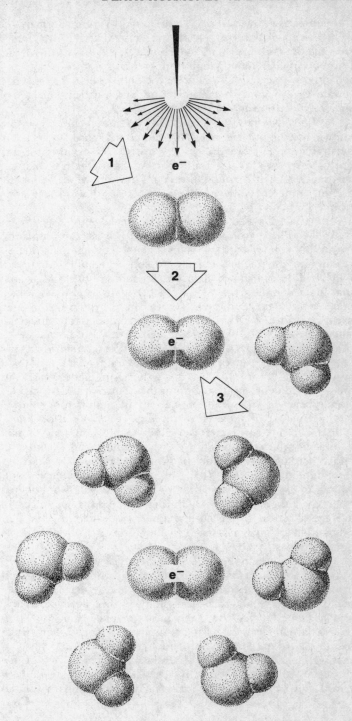

### Negative air ions.

"Air ion" is the term authors and researchers apply to a group of specific chemical entities that result when ionization occurs in air. This vague term has not encouraged the wide acceptance of air ions as an important biological factor. There is evidence now that one specific molecule may be responsible for many of the observed biological effects. That molecule is the hydrated superoxide radical anion $(O_2^-)(H_2O)_n$ with $n$ having values in the range 4 to 8. It is formed when (1) an ordinary oxygen molecule combines with a free electron to form (2) the superoxide radical anion. (3) The anion is then surrounded by water molecules, which tend to stabilize it. In high concentrations the superoxide is effective in killing bacteria; lower concentrations are thought to bring about therapeutic effects in humans.

nucleus and an equal number of negatively charged electrons surrounding these. Electrons, however, are 1,800 times lighter than protons, and, under various circumstances, can slip away from the atom's grasp. When this happens the atom becomes positively charged. If, on the other hand, an electrically balanced atom attracts a stray electron, the atom becomes negatively charged. Under most natural conditions, the air around us contains between one and two thousand ions per cubic centimeter, in a ratio of five positive ions to every four negative ones. These proportions may fluctuate slightly at certain times, and can vary radically under particular circumstances.

We are all familiar with some manifestations of disbalanced atmospheric ionization, such as static electricity, and thunder and lightning (which is the electrical discharge between a large mass of positive ions in the air and the negative charge in the earth). At least as far back as the eighteenth century, many learned men were aware of atmospheric electricity. Around the same time that Benjamin Franklin was conducting his famous experiments to attempt to capture this force, others, such as L'Abbé Nollet, and Father Giam Battista Baccaria of the University of Turin, Italy, were finding evidence that atmospheric electricity is essential to the health of plant life, and possibly also to that of humans and animals. But it was not until the end of the nineteenth century that scientists understood that this electricity results from ionized gases.

Since then, there has been a very gradual accumulation of knowledge about this phenomenon and its effects on living organisms. Krueger and Smith have contributed much to our more recent knowledge in this field. For one thing, they found that an excess of positive ions can cause an overproduction of serotonin in mice, displaying itself first as hyperactivity, then soon as exhaustion, anxiety, and depression. They also found that large dosages of negative ions can reverse the response and have a calming effect by reducing the amount of serotonin in the brain and other tissues. [186]

After learning of the link Krueger and Smith had discovered between ions and serotonin, Sulman enlisted meteorologists and physicists to help him measure ion levels in the air during the Sharav. They found that two days before the wind arrives, the ion count more than doubles, and the proportion of positive ions far exceeds that of negative ions. Apparently, the dry wind blowing across the desert sands generates static electricity. This breeds a preponderance of positive ions, while the flying dust particles attract and bind much of the existing negative ions. The electrical front is pushed forward by the atmospheric pressures that produce the wind, and it arrives before the air currents. It is always two days before the wind comes that weather-sensitive people experi-

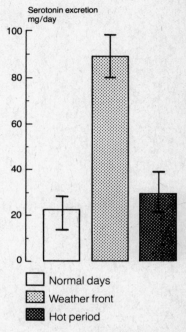

Serotonin excretion mg/day

☐ Normal days
▨ Weather front
■ Hot period

*Weather and serotonin production.*
Weather-sensitive patients studied by Sulman showed many significant biochemical changes in response to specific weather changes. Sulman suggests that the air-ion fluctuations associated with the arrival of the Sharav are responsible for many of the biochemical responses. The change in serotonin excretion is one of the more dramatic changes. Since the daily excretion of serotonin indicates the amount the body makes, it appears that the arrival of the Sharav causes an overproduction of serotonin.

ence the greatest discomfort. The wind itself may actually help sweep away the sick air.

Armed with a better understanding of the Sharav phenomenon, Sulman began an intensive ten-year study of its effects on the human system. By 1971, he was able to conclude that there are three separate physical responses to the Sharav.

First, there is an overproduction of serotonin in the brain and other organs, which may result in anxiety, tension, nausea, hot flashes, pains around the heart, migraine, depression, breathing difficulties, and aggravation of bronchial problems. Serotonin irritation can also lead to overproduction of histamines, which is why Sharav victims often feel like they have colds.

Second, the excess of serotonin may initially activate the production of large quantities of adrenalin and noradrenalin. At

Serotonin hyperproduction:
Irritation syndrome
(Urinary serotonin and 5-HIAA increased)
215 patients

Adrenal deficiency:
Exhaustion syndrome
(Urinary adrenaline, noradrenaline, 17-KS, 17-OH decreased)
220 patients

Hyperthyroidism
"Forme Fruste"
(Urinary thyroxine and histamine increased, serotonin sometimes increased)
65 patients

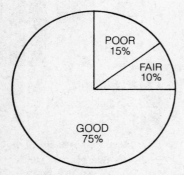
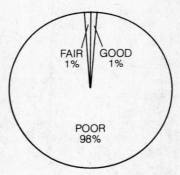
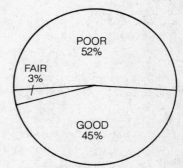

Sleeplessness, irritability, tension, electrified hair, migraine, vomiting, swelling, rheumatic pain in scars, muscles, and joints, palpitations, precordial pain, flushes with sweat or chills, runny nose, sore throat, vertigo, tremor, oversensitivity to light, sound, smells

Hypotension, fatigue, apathy, blackout, depression, confusion, hypoglycaemic spells

Asomnia, irritability, tension, vomiting, palpitations, precordial pain, sweat, tremor, abdominal pain, diarrhea, allergic reactions, overactivity, fatigue, depression, confusion

*Negative air ionization as a treatment for heat-stress symptoms.*

Sulman has been researching the connection between weather sensitivity, biochemical changes, and negative air ions. Elevated serotonin levels during weather fronts are among the many changes he noticed. In a study of 500 weather-sensitive female patients, Sulman identified three types of reactions to heat stress in his patients. He then evaluated the effectiveness of negative air ionization in treating the symptoms. The study was done "double blind": neither the subject nor the researcher knew who specifically was receiving the treatment. The pie graphs represent the three syndromes; the degree of improvement by negative air ionization is indicated by good, fair, or poor. The per cent improvement is represented by the segment of the circle.

first, these will make a person feel stimulated and euphoric, but after a few years the exhausted adrenal system can no longer produce enough hormones to maintain normal energy levels, and a state of exhaustion will set in. The same thing happens with long-term abuse of stimulant drugs.

Third, the thyroid becomes overactivated. This causes symptoms similar to those of serotonin irritation, such as tension, anxiety, and high histamine production. [155]

The conclusion drawn from most research is that excessive amounts of positive ions are generally unhealthy, whereas abundant quantities of negative ions are usually beneficial. Even when humans or animals are exposed to extraordinarily large doses of negative ions, no harm occurs. But when there is a complete absence of any kind of ions in the environment, serious damage can result.

Several decades before either Sulman or Krueger began their research on ions, Soviet scientist A. L. Tchijewsky had made some remarkable discoveries about their effects on living organisms. Tchijewsky kept mice, rats, guinea pigs, and rabbits in totally deionized air. Nearly all the animals were dead within two weeks. Autopsies revealed fatty liver, kidney failure, degeneration of heart muscle, and anemia. These were mostly due to the improper utilization of oxygen. Other experiments have shown that an excess of positive ions can also impair oxygenation of the blood and the ability of the body to utilize oxygen. An overdose of positive ions may reduce breathing capacity by as much as 30 per cent. On the other hand, large doses of negative ions improve the blood's oxygenation and the body's use of oxygen. [381]

Another Soviet scientist, D. A. Lapitsky, kept laboratory animals in oxygen-deficient air until they were on the verge of asphyxiation, then suffused their environment with negative ions. The animals recovered immediately. [348]

During the mid-1940s, a third Soviet researcher, A. A. Minkh, conducted a series of ion experiments on athletes. He had them lift weights to the point of exhaustion. The ones who were given large doses of negative ions recovered first. Those given overdoses of mixed positive and negative ions were second, and those who breathed normal air recovered last. He also tested endurance gains under various ionic conditions. The subjects practiced daily running in place until collapse, and their improvement in endurance time at the end of one month was noted. Those breathing normal air improved no more than 24 per cent, but those breathing negatively ionized air improved more than ten times that much. The gains made by the latter group were retained for about ten days after they had been returned to a normally ionized environment, and then gradually tapered off. [348]

The lungs are affected by ions in other ways also. The respiratory tract is lined with microscopic hairs called cilia, which maintain a lashing motion of about fifteen beats per second to

*Serotonin*

sweep foreign particles, such as dust and pollen, away from the lungs. Ion starvation or overdoses of positive ions will slow the cilial movement to as few as ten beats per second and greatly reduce their efficiency, but large doses of negative ions can rapidly restore normal activity and even raise it to twenty beats per second.[348, 349]

The sun's ultraviolet rays, the radioactivity within the Earth, and, to some extent, vegetation are the major natural sources of ions in the atmosphere. More ions are generated on a sunny day than when it is cloudy. There are usually more ions in a forest than in a field. Plants take up ions from the earth, which is negatively charged, and emit them from the tips of their leaves. The description which we have already given of normal air (1,000 to 2,000 ions per cc., 5 pos to 4 neg) is typical of a sunny day in the country. In cities the ion balance is often five positive to one negative, and sometimes the total ion count may be close to zero. The "unnatural" nature of the city is entirely to blame for this. Steel and concrete tend to absorb negative ions. The friction of moving vehicles against the air generates positive ions, while the positively charged metal bodies of the autos attract and trap the beneficial negative ions. A similar thing happens when static electricity is generated by rubbing certain materials together, or by walking in footwear on a woolen or synthetic carpet.[350]

In buildings with central heating and sealed air-conditioning systems, the ion condition is even worse. Air filters trap ions, especially negative ones. The movement of air currents through the metal ducts of ventilator shafts also captures negative ions while generating positive ones. A man-made miniature Sharav is created in buildings that contain such systems.[350]

The Sharav and similar wind-related ion disturbances are produced by the friction of air currents over dry lands. Wherever sufficient moisture is present, these imbalances do not occur. That is why sea breezes are refreshing and invigorating, and desert winds are enervating. Healthful negative ions are also generated during the breaking up of water into fine droplets. High negative-ion counts can be found near breaking waves and ocean spray, fountains, and waterfalls. The total ion count of the air around Niagara Falls can run as high as 100,000 ions per cubic centimeter, and these are predominantly of negative charge.[351]

Pollen in the air traps negative ions just as the dry desert dust does. When the pollen count is high, there may be a sharp imbalance in atmospheric ionization. Since this electrical condition can increase histamine production, it can add to the woes of those already suffering from hay fever. The friction of machinery also generates positive ions and traps negative ones. So do many kinds of electrical and electronic equipment. Computers, TV sets, and radar units are among the worst offenders.

People often feel drained and out of sorts after spending an hour or so at the laundromat. In busy laundromats the air may contain large quantities of positive ions and be almost depleted of negative ions. The friction created by the tumbling of dried clothing in hot, dry air against the rotating metal drums of the dryers generates huge amounts of static electricity and sickens the air. Even our clothing, while we wear it, can do this to a great extent. Most fabrics (wools, silks, and synthetics) will produce a static charge when they are rubbed together. Cotton, linen, and hemp fiber are almost the only exceptions. Just the friction of electrogenic materials against the air, or rustling against themselves as we move, can trap negative ions around the body and generate positive ions. Some ion-sensitive people have benefited from wearing only cotton or linen clothing.

On a pleasant spring day in 1978, several members of the Megahealth Society and I visited the Tutankhamen exhibit at the Los Angeles County Museum of Art. Our spirits were elated when we entered the museum, but within minutes we began to feel oppressed and exhausted. We had no idea why, and even jested that King Tut's curse had returned. Later that evening, however, we met several other people who had seen the exhibit a few weeks earlier and had had the same enervating experience. Suddenly I realized the cause of the mysterious malaise and felt foolish for not having guessed it sooner. To protect the priceless relics from deterioration, the atmospheric conditions of Egypt had to be duplicated. The air in the museum chambers was maintained at exactly 70°F with no humidity. Hundreds of people, most of them wearing synthetic fabrics, moved continuously through these rooms, brushing against each other and generating a static charge that depleted the air of its negative ions and filled it with positive ones. We had all been the temporary victims of a synthetic Hamsin.

One of the most noticeable causes of ion alterations in nature is the electrical storm. Humans and animals become tense as a storm gathers, because the air is becoming positively charged. The release of this charge as lightning generates large amounts of negative ions and restores electrostatic equilibrium. Tension then subsides. Some people always seem to know when foul weather is approaching. "I can feel it in my bones," they say. This is not clairvoyance; it is simply the ionic imbalance that precedes a storm, causing a rise in serotonin that irritates the body's sensitive spots. Old injuries act up. Arthritis, rheumatism, stiff joints, and the many aches and pains that often accompany old age become more pronounced.

Warm, dry south winds and lightning storms are not the only natural phenomena that cause imbalances in atmospheric electricity. A similar imbalance is caused by the moon. Ranging between 25 and 250 miles above the Earth is a layer of charged particles known as the ionosphere. One of its functions is to help maintain a normal ion balance in the Earth's atmosphere. The upper portion of the ionosphere is negatively charged, the lower

## Air Ions

In 1958, Hungarian scientist J. M. Barnothy housed a group of aging mice within magnetic fields for periods of from one to four weeks. The results were that the mice appeared younger, were 30 per cent more active, acquired immunity to cancer metastases, and experienced regression of breast-cancer transplants.

portion positively charged. The moon, like the Earth, is negatively charged. When it is closer to the Earth, its negative charge repels the negative ions of the upper ionosphere, and these, in turn, push some of the lower ionosphere's positive ions into our immediate atmosphere, where they cause erratic behavior in some humans and animals.[349]

Dr. Norman Shealy, neurosurgeon and head of the Pain Clinic at La Crosse, Wisconsin, recently made a survey among other surgeons and learned that 80 per cent of excessive bleeding in surgical patients takes place when the moon is full. In each of the explanations for this phenomenon offered so far, positive ions are implicated in some way, if not entirely blamed. Overproduction of serotonin may also be involved. As was mentioned earlier, surgeons in southern Europe have noticed the same bleeding problem when the Föhn condition prevails.[349]

It has also been observed that the full moon can hasten birth if pregnancy is near termination. This is because serotonin functions as an oxytocic, stimulating contractions of the uterus and hastening parturition. It was Felix Sulman's studies of the role of serotonin in pregnancy that led to his discoveries about atmospheric polarity. He had found that pregnant rats abort when injected with serotonin. Sulman gave drugs that stimulate the production of serotonin to twenty pregnant women who were scheduled for legal abortions. Each of them aborted spontaneously. He later reversed the procedure by giving serotonin inhibitors to women who could not remain pregnant. Nearly all were able to give birth successfully.[349]

Although positive ions can induce labor by stimulating serotonin production, their noxious traits can be a threat to the well-being and survival of both mother and child at the crucial moment of birth. For this reason, negative-ion generators are now being used in the delivery and recovery rooms of some Swiss hospitals. Both Russian and Italian scientists have also found that negative ions can promote the flow of milk in lactating mothers if production is below par, but no increase occurs when lactation is already sufficient.[349]

In many other ways, negative ions are finding their way into modern medicine. In Great Britain they are now being used in migraine therapy. They have also been used at Philadelphia's Northeastern General Hospital in the treatment of serious burns. Because of the stress and shock that the body suffers from burn injuries, there is a sudden increase in the release of serotonin. This heightens sensitivity to pain and inhibits healing. Large dosages of negative ions promote tissue repair, lessen likelihood of infection, reduce pain and discomfort, tranquilize the patient, and minimize scarring.[349]

Negative ions are also valuable in treating allergies, sinus conditions, and respiratory complaints. An ion-therapy section was installed in a factory in Meissen, East Germany, for workers exposed to occupational pulmonary hazards. The healthful feelings that the men experienced from the treatments prompted many of them to ask permission to bring their families. Soon, local physicians were sending bronchial cases to the factory for therapy.

Recently, a link has even been found between ions and cancer. Clarence D. Cone, working for NASA, discovered that normal cells carry a negative surface charge that becomes greatly reduced during malignancy.[46] The U.S. National Cancer Institute is now studying the possibility of ion therapy as a treatment for cancer. In the Soviet Union, the use of strongly ionized air on mice with transplanted cancers resulted in reduction of the malignancy within six weeks. The mice that received ion therapy lived long beyond the untreated controls.[349] In Chapter 6 it was mentioned that vitamin $B_3$ also places a negative charge on the blood-cell surface, and thereby increases the cell's oxygen-carrying ability. The improved oxygenation that occurs in a negative-ion environment could be explained by this surface charge. Perhaps the vitamin and the ions could work synergistically in this respect to further protect against cancer and senile degeneration.

There is another important role of ion treatments in dealing with cancer. Large amounts of serotonin accumulate around malignant tumors and increase sensitivity to pain.[263] Opiates, standardly given to terminal patients, lose their effectiveness long before the end is near. Even when there is no chance of saving a patient, negative ions should be administered to relieve the serotonin-induced torment, and make the victim more comfortable.

From all that we have said about negative ions, it is obvious that they must have many medical and remedial applications. Because large doses of negative ions improve oxygenation, physicians might find them useful in cases of carbon-monoxide poisoning and gangrene. To further their effectiveness in these situations, they could be given in conjunction with vitamins $B_3$, $B_{15}$, A, and E. Since the brain requires oxygen-rich blood to function properly, negative ions might also be used to enhance learning. The positive-ion poisoning and negative-ion starvation induced by the central heating systems in some of our school buildings may be retarding many an otherwise promising student whose only problem is ion sensitivity.

It has also been observed that negative ions improve the body's ability to assimilate vitamin C.[348] It is possible that some infection cases that do not respond satisfactorily to ascorbic-acid therapy fail only because of poor absorption. Perhaps Linus Pauling and his colleagues could synergize the effectiveness of this vitamin with negative ions in their megascorbic treatments of cancer, influenza, and the common cold.[260, 261, 262]

Negative ions may even be helpful in treating certain forms of schizophrenia and other biochemically rooted psychoses. A number of links have been found between serotonin and mental

Tryptophan

5-Hydroxytryptophan

Serotonin

MAO-regulated step

5-Hydroxyindole acetaldehyde

5-Hydroxyindole acetic acid

*Pathway of serotonin biosynthesis and degradation.*

disorders.[409, 410] Increasing the brain-serotonin levels in dogs produces gross behavioral changes.[142] People with mental disease often have a high indole concentration in their urine.[353, 354] This indicates an overproduction of serotonin. Although we don't know whether abnormal serotonin production is a cause or a symptom of the problem, ion therapy could probably offer some relief to many mentally disturbed persons.

## Antiserotonin Drugs

Serotonin is an indole-based substance that is a biogenic amine in both the general and the psychopharmacological senses, since it is an amine synthesized from normal dietary precursors, and is involved in the functioning of neurons. It was first isolated from intestinal cells (argentaffin cells of the gastric mucous membrane) in 1937 by V. Erspamer, who also demonstrated that it is a smooth-muscle stimulant. It is also found in other tissues, bound with various substances, such as histamine and heparin, and stored within the cytoplasmic granules of the cells. In 1947, I. H. Page showed it to be a pressor substance in clotted blood, and, in 1953, to be present in the brain. It is also stored in the vesicles of the nerve endings, and is discretely released as needed for nerve-impulse transmission. It occurs in a bound state in the blood platelets. When these break up during clotting, serotonin is released, and helps prevent bleeding by constricting blood vessels around the injury.[57] Excessive bleeding during a full moon or ion wind is apparently caused not by serotonin, but perhaps by the anticoagulant heparin released in the breaking of serotonin/heparin complexes.

Serotonin occurs in vegetables as well as animals, and is found in some edible plants. There are large amounts of it in unripe bananas. Matoke, a species of banana that is eaten green, is the dietary staple of many Africans. There is no harm in eating unripe bananas occasionally, but when they are consumed as heavily as they are by some African peoples, free serotonin levels in the system may rise dangerously and can result in cardiovascular stress. This is doubtlessly the reason that endomyocardial fibrosis is a common disease among matoke eaters. In 1962, M. A. Crawford in East Africa, and J. M. Foy with J. R. Parrot in West Africa, showed that circulating serotonin levels in matoke eaters are three to fifteen times higher than normal.[50, 102]

Serotonin is synthesized in the body from the essential amino acid tryptophan; first by a hydroxylase enzyme that converts it to 5-hydroxytryptophan (5-HTP); and then by a decarboxylase enzyme, to form 5-hydroxytryptamine (5-HT), which is the proper name for serotonin. Excessive amounts of serotonin are broken down (deaminated) to 5-hydroxyindole acetaldehyde by monoamine oxidase (MAO), and this aldehyde is then oxidized by aldehyde dehydrogenase to form 5-hydroxyindole acetic acid (5-HIAA), which is readily excreted through the kidneys. Only circulating serotonin, which is not bound inertly to other substances or stored in vesicles, is subject to deamination and excretion. Stored or bound, it does not react.[184] Researchers Paolo Timiras and Paul Segall have some evidence which agrees with existing reports that levels of serotonin in some specific brain regions rise with age. They also discovered that, at the same time, dopamine levels go down.[315]

Dopamine is a biogenic catecholamine, properly known as 3-hydroxytyramine. It is formed enzymatically in the body, first by the hydrolysis of tyrosine to dopa, and then by the decarboxylation of dopa to dopamine. Dopa is properly known as 3-hydroxytyrosine, or, more accurately, beta-3,4-dihydroxyphenylalanine, for (part of) which the letters DOPA are an acronym. Dopamine is a precursor for another and perhaps more well-known catecholamine, norepinephrine.

Besides the many dangers and unpleasant symptoms from excessive amounts of serotonin described in this chapter, this neurohormone has also been implicated as one of the substances involved in triggering the "death hormone" response of the hypothalamus and pituitary. Timiras and Segall have been developing evidence that this is so. Earlier, we mentioned how these two workers more or less duplicated Clive McCay's calorie-restriction experiments by limiting the essential amino acid tryptophan in the diets of immature animals. It would seem, as with McCay, that their success in extending the lives of these creatures was entirely due to a delay of maturation, and that the only portion of life than can be extended by this technique is the period between infancy and puberty. But Timiras and Segall believe that their results may have been partly brought about because the synthesis of serotonin was inhibited by restriction of its amino-acid precursor. They are interested in exploring whether they can also extend the period of life after puberty by similarly limiting the availability of tryptophan. Some of their experiments indicate that this may be possible.

Timiras and Segall, wanting to find out whether the life-extending results of their tryptophan-restriction experiments were merely due to a delay in maturity, fed two rats a completely normal diet until the animals were thirteen months old. The diet was then made tryptophan-deficient, and was maintained as such until the rats were 26 months old. The diet was then normalized again. The animals showed some signs of rejuvenation. When shaved, for instance, their hair grew back faster than that of the controls. The appearance of their coats was better than normal for their age, but after three months, its condition had degenerated and was about the same as that of the controls. At 40 months, one of the rats was still alive, but so were a few of the controls. Other experiments with calorie restriction at middle life have yielded more or less similar results. The general conclusion is that dietary

*Tyrosine*

*L-DOPA*

*Dopamine*

*Norepinephrine*

*Pathway of dopamine and norepinephrine biosynthesis.*

"A model system is proposed which suggests that aging involves a genetically programmed process encoded within specific regions of the central nervous system and is characterized by a gradual ascendency of inhibitory over excitatory influences."

Paul E. Segall

restrictions commenced after puberty can somewhat rejuvenate the immune system, but do not appear to bring about any significant increases in lifespan.[331]

Despite the inconclusiveness of most experiments, many gerontologists believe that techniques for decreasing serotonin, especially in the brain, still hold immense promise for life extension, even after puberty. But depriving the body of an amino acid essential to health and growth seems to be a rather haphazard approach. Tryptophan has other functions than in the formation of protein and the synthesis of serotonin. For one thing, it is a precursor of niacin, and it is now well-known that some individuals need as much of this vitamin as they can get.

Can high tryptophan diets or the high serotonin intake of the matoke eaters hasten the release of "death hormones"? If so, can avoidance of excessive dietary tryptophan and serotonin delay the "death hormone" response?

Although it may lead to early death from cardiovascular stress, dietary serotonin is unlikely to hasten the release of hypothalamic "death hormones." Ingested serotonin will enter the bloodstream and, if excessive, may endanger the muscle and blood vessels of the heart, but little if any will pass through the membranous barrier between the bloodstream and the brain. Precursors of serotonin can cross the barrier, but serotonin itself cannot.[155] Any serotonin in the brain had to be manufactured there. Under normal circumstances, most of the body's serotonin is bound with other materials or stored in granules, and is released in minute quantities, only as needed; or excessively during stress. It is conceivable that a person could have enough free serotonin in the hypothalamic regions to trigger "death hormones," yet have low serum levels of it. One could also have high amounts in the blood and low amounts in the brain. Hence the total amount of serotonin in the body is not necessarily a pertinent factor in the sequences that influence "death hormone" release.

On the other hand, Timiras and Segall have demonstrated that the amounts of tryptophan in the diet may be reflected in the amounts of free serotonin in both the bloodstream and the brain. They have also shown that severe tryptophan restriction is too hazardous to be of any practical value for self-experimenting longevists. It is possible, though, that limiting tryptophan intake to only the amount required for normal health, and obtaining vitamin B3 as dietary and supplemental niacin or niacinamide, may help keep down the amounts of serotonin in the blood and brain. A worthwhile study might be to establish a diet that provides just enough tryptophan, and to find out exactly how much influence this has on hypthalamic serotonin. Even if it does help, there is still the problem of preventing the conditions that cause excessive conversion of tryptophan to serotonin. There may, however, already be several solutions to this problem.

Earlier in this section, we discussed the influence of atmospheric ions on serotonin levels. Among the many beneficial effects of high negative and low positive ionization are that it raises the amount of dopamine, and lowers the amount of serotonin, in both the blood and the brain. The relationship between ionization, serotonin, and aging (and health, in general) demands extensive research. Atmospheric-ion manipulation is certain to be a means of preventing the known and proven damages from overproduction of serotonin, and may offer a method of slowing down one of the biological aging clocks.

In March of 1978, at the Alcor Life-Extension Conference in Los Angeles, I asked Dr. Segall if he had considered the connections between air ions, serotonin, and life extension. He said that he had, and would like to see someone explore it experimentally. Perhaps, as general awareness of the ion phenomenon expands, he and other workers may find more support for research in this area.

I also asked Dr. Segall if he had considered the experimental use of drugs, such as PCPA (parachlorphenalanine), which interfere with the enzymatic conversion of tryptophan to serotonin.[184] He told me that he is using this drug on animals, but it has many toxic side effects. PCPA—not to be confused with PCP (phencyclidine)—is apparently not the ideal drug for controlling hypothalamic serotonin and inhibiting the secretion of "death hormone"–releasing factors. Still, there are one or two other known drugs which may prove useful.

## DOPAMINE PRECURSORS

The disorder known as parkinsonism, or Parkinson's disease, involves low concentrations of dopamine in the brain.[162] Because dopamine will not pass through the blood-brain barrier, oral doses or injections of it are useless for treating this disorder. But dopa, its precursor, readily passes from the bloodstream to the brain, where it is converted to dopamine. It is the levorotary or *l* forms of dopa and dopamine that are biologically active, which is why Levodopa and L-dopa are the names commonly used for this drug.

We have already mentioned that amounts of dopamine in the system go down when those of serotonin go up, and vice versa. Large amounts of serotonin in the brain can interfere with normal appetites for food and sex. Many cases of impotence in the male, or lack of desire in either gender, result from having too much serotonin and too little dopamine. Such a condition is usually the result of prolonged stress, worry, overwork, poor nutrition, negative-ion starvation, or positive-ion poisoning. Many older parkinsonism patients receiving L-dopa have experienced strong sexual urges. This fact has led some writers to suggest that L-dopa is a sex stimulant or aphrodisiac, which it is

*L-DOPA*

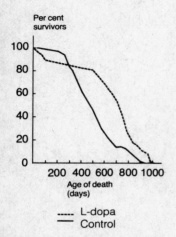

Per cent
survivors

```
100
 80
 60
 40
 20
  0
    200 400 600 800 1000
```
Age of death
(days)

----- L-dopa
——— Control

*L-dopa prolongs the lifespan of mice.*

L-dopa is being consumed by many persons with Parkinson's disease. While evaluating some effects of long-term L-dopa consumption, Cotzias noted a life-extension effect on mice. The maximum lifespan was increased slightly, but the mean lifespan was increased up to 50 per cent. The results shown here are for mice fed L-dopa as 4 per cent of their food; farm animals have been raised on velvet beans, which have a 13 per cent L-dopa content.

The change in the shape of the survival curve with the L-dopa diet suggests there is a decrease in the incidence of diseases which kill animals before they reach their maximum possible age. This could result from a stimulation of the immune system by the L-dopa diet.

not. Concupiscence (or horniness, if you prefer) is a natural state for healthy humans of most ages. Sadly, such destructive forces as guilt, repression, fear, worry, tension, and general stress can incite overproduction of serotonin and diminish otherwise healthy appetites. Except for this, there is usually no physical reason why men and women should not have almost as much sexual desire in old age as they had in youth.

Healthy libido is not the only aspect of youthfulness that L-dopa can effect. At Michigan State University, Joseph Meites used it to induce ovulation in aging female rats that had long since ceased ovulating.[309] Hence, in addition to retarding some aspects of aging, the drug may actually reverse others.

In 1974, George C. Cotzias, at Brookhaven National Laboratory in New York, extended both the prime of life and the total lifespan of mice by feeding them large dosages of L-dopa. He also reported that initial tests with the drug on humans showed no harmful side effects.[47] Observers have noted that some parkinsonism patients who have been taking L-dopa for many years appear to be retaining youthful characteristics somewhat better than normal. But it is still too soon to leap to any conclusions.

L-dopa is generally available only by prescription as a treatment for Parkinson's disease. A person cannot purchase tablets of it from a pharmacy without written medical authorization, and it is unlikely that a physician would be willing to prescribe it as a longevity drug or for any reason other than parkinsonism. Still, it is not a completely controlled substance. It can be bought in powdered form from some chemical supply houses for about $150 a pound. But it is not as easy to obtain chemicals from suppliers as it was a few years ago. The federal government has placed many restrictions and liabilities on chemical companies, and most are hesitant to sell to anyone except established laboratories and other legitimate groups.

Some self-experimenting longevists who have been able to obtain L-dopa have been taking it for several years. They report favorable results with no ill effects. The numerous instances cited in the medical literature of parkinsonism patients who experience unwanted side effects from the drug probably result from the size of the therapeutic dosage, which is between four and six grams daily, taken in three or more divided doses. Most longevists use less than half these amounts. The *Physicians' Desk Reference* lists at least a hundred adverse reactions to L-dopa, including nausea, anorexia, vomiting, gas, aggravation of existing ulcer, diarrhea, constipation, dizziness, lethargy, insomnia, nightmares, blurred vision, numbness of extremities, tremor, headache, dry mouth, involuntary movements, rash, and cardiac irregularities. Most of these are fairly rare. The minor gastric problems are somewhat more common, but usually only early in treatment. They are easily relieved by temporarily reducing the dosage. Persistence of the more serious reactions may indicate that the patient should discontinue the drug. Titration of dosage is almost always practiced, starting with a total daily intake of 500 to 1,000 mg, in divided doses, and increasing by 100 mg every three or four days until optimum dosage is reached. Patients are usually advised to take the drug with meals to minimize the possibility of side effects.

Persons with active peptic ulcer, narrow-angle glaucoma, bronchial asthma, emphysema, and renal, hepatic, or endocrinal disorders should be cautious about using L-dopa. The drug increases both the pharmacological effects and the toxicity of MAO inhibitors. People who take these should not use L-dopa, even in the lesser antiaging doses, except under the care of a physician. The same goes for people with psychoses or severe psychoneuroses (unfavorable mental changes may occur), and for anyone with a history of myocardial infarction with residual arrhythmias. [291]

Several researchers report that 10 to 25 mg of pyridoxine (vitamin B6) will quickly neutralize most side effects of L-dopa. Unfortunately, it also reduces the medical effectiveness of the drug and probably its life-extending properties as well. [88, 165, 289] Physicians are advised not to prescribe multivitamin preparations during L-dopa therapy. Carl Pfeiffer of the Bio Brain Center finds, however, that the vitamin does not interfere with the drug if zinc intake is adequate. [270]

Recently, a new form of the antiparkinsonism drug has become available. It bears the trade name Sinemet and is a mixture of ten parts L-dopa and one part carbidopa. One of the problems with L-dopa is that much of it is converted into dopamine in the bloodstream before it can enter the brain. Carbidopa inhibits the decarboxylation of aromatic amino acids like L-dopa. This allows more of the drug to reach the brain, where it can be converted into dopamine. Because of this, lower, less-toxic dosages of L-dopa can be given. As a serotonin-control drug for delaying the triggered release of the "death hormone," Sinemet holds even greater promise than straight L-dopa. Also, vitamin B6 does not interfere with the drug when carbidopa is present. There are fewer contraindications and side effects with Sinemet, mainly because of the lower dosage. Nursing mothers are advised not to use it. A person who has been taking L-dopa should stop for two months before commencing with Sinemet. [234]

## PSYCHEDELICS
During the late 1950s and early 1960s, several researchers were trying to discover the precise mechanisms and pathways by which LSD-25 and other psychedelic drugs bring about their spectacular alterations in thought and perception. Several experiments led to the hypothesis that it was, at least in part, the antiserotonin properties of these drugs that caused the mental changes. [410] An assumption was making the rounds at that time—

"The days of our years are threescore and ten; and if by reason of strength, they be fourscore years, yet is their strength labor and sorrow; for it is cut off, and we fly away."

*Psalms* 90:10

frequently among those who felt it necessary to defend their use of these drugs—that LSD and other psychotropic substances could lessen the harmful effects of serotonin. This notion gained some support in 1962, when R. D. Bunag and E. J. Walaszek demonstrated that lysergic-acid derivatives blocked the arterial-pressure response to serotonin, histamine, and adrenaline.[34] Some years later, Denckla, Guillemin, Timiras, Segall, and others began to develop and explore the concept that a "death hormone" may be triggered in the brain by a specific combination of conditions, one of them being the accumulation of high concentrations of serotonin.[124, 312] Word of their ideas and efforts trickled down among the ranks of longevists, some of whom, already being psychedelic consumers, began to cultivate the belief that the steadfast, lifelong use of LSD could inhibit serotonin's action so much that it would delay release of this "hormone." Many even misconstrued that the drug would act by lowering serotonin levels.

None of these lysergic longevists had an educated guess about the dosage needed to derive this benefit, or how often it must be taken. But since they were already using the drug for its mental manifestations, they were naturally glad to have an additional justification for their use of a socially and legally condemned drug, and, at the same time, to be able to entertain a glimpse of hope that the brief years of their mortal lives might stretch a bit beyond the average human ration of three score and ten. Most of them, of course, had enough respect for their minds and bodies not to embark on psychedelic excursions more often than once every month or so. Yet it was obvious that the short-lasting serotonin-blocking action of the mind drugs is unlikely to extend life much when they are taken so infrequently. Some self-experimenters attempted to resolve the dilemma by taking small daily dosages, not enough to produce any psychedelic effects. Many people had already discovered that ingesting small, subthreshold quantities of psychedelics, especially psilocybe mushrooms and peyote, gave them a general feeling of well-being.

Although I believe that psychoactive drugs have valid uses for personal enlightenment and psychotherapy, the evidence at hand strongly suggests that they possess no life-extending properties. In fact, there is even some evidence that habitual use of many of these drugs could shorten life, especially if a serotonin-induced "death hormone" actually exists.

It has been established that LSD, psilocybin, and many other psychoactive chemicals* briefly block the action of sero-

---

* These include DMT (dimethyltryptamine), yohimbine, ibogaine, harmine-related alkaloids from yage (*Banisteriopsis caapi*), ALD-52 (acetyllysergic acid diethylamide), and MLD-41 (methyllysergic acid diethylamide). *Cannabis* (marijuana and hashish) does not have this effect, although it might slow down the rate at which serotonin builds up if it were to reduce stress.

tonin in many tissues. [152, 155, 156, 157] But since these drugs are
indoles, they also inhibit MAO. When the MAO enzyme is
blocked, serotonin is not broken down to 5-HIAA and will accumulate in the tissues. Furthermore, since neurohormones cannot
be deactivated before they have carried out their functions, any
serotonin whose action is blocked will remain in the tissues
unaltered.

In 1962, D. X. Freedman and N. J. Giarman found that
LSD slightly elevated the amounts of serotonin in the brains of
dogs. [106] In 1963, Freedman measured the amount of serotonin in
the brains of rats and rabbits after they had been given LSD, and
found it up by 17 per cent. Similar increases occurred with
psilocybin, ALD-52, and MLD-41. [107] Around the same time,
D. V. S. Sankar and others administered radioactive 5-HTP (the
immediate precursor of serotonin) to rabbits, followed 45 minutes
later by an effective dose of LSD. By tracing the radioactive precursor, they were able to conclude that LSD increases serotonin
everywhere in the brain except the cerebrum and cerebellum. [324]

We need not cite the many lurid press reports of nightmare
trips, drug-induced suicides, and human vegetables who never
recovered, to see that there are some unwanted side effects from
the excessive use of psychoactive drugs. There is some evidence
that LSD and similar drugs temporarily increase the permeability
of the BBB, and that this change may play some role in the
psychedelic experience. Substances that are released into the
bloodstream by these drugs could reach the brain while this
permeable state prevails. Other substances, harmless in the blood
but not in the brain, may also reach this organ at the time. [151]
Unfortunately, because of restrictive laws and social attitudes,
research on psychedelic drugs — except by the military as
weapons — has virtually come to a standstill.

There may be another clue about psychoactive indoles and
aging in the folk-wisdom of the Indians of central Mexico. A
*curandero* (healer) will often share a dose of psilocybe mushrooms
with his patient. Bonded, for the moment, by this sacrament, the
two can delve into the nature of the ailment and diagnose its
spiritual or psychic causes. For the patient such an experience
may be rare, but for the *curandero* it is more likely to be a regular
duty. Many *curanderos* have noted that this frequent ingestion of
the magic mushroom promotes early aging, and will not take the
mushroom with the patient. [220] Gerontologists in search of the
elusive "death hormone" might do well to take a closer look at this
phenomenon.

---

Mind drugs as powerful as LSD and psilocybin are not toys.
They are tools. Like any tool, they have their time, place, and
purpose. They must be used with knowledge and skill if anything
*continued*

worthy is to come from their use, and should be employed only in the tasks for which they are designed. A trained carpenter would not indiscriminately substitute a wrench and screwdriver for a hammer and chisel. Nor would it be wise to put an electric saw in the hands of someone who had not yet learned to manage it. Most of us do not properly understand the various uses of the many psychotropic tools available today. However, it is improbable that they can extend lifespan by blocking serotonin.

## PRACTICAL APPLICATIONS

Whether there is or is not a serotonin-induced "death hormone," it is certain that excessive serotonin has many debilitating effects on the body that could lead to early demise. Amounts of serotonin can be controlled with divided daily doses of L-dopa or Sinemet, but we cannot recommend self-treatment with these drugs. Furthermore, it is not easy to obtain them without a prescription.

Some longevists have thought about eating a diet that is high in dopa, which is found in some plants used for food. An exceptionally rich source is the velvet bean (*Stizolobium deeringianum*), an annual legume often used as stock feed in the southern U.S.A. The dried bean contains about 13 per cent L-dopa. [48]

Avoiding stress and poorly ionized areas helps curb abnormal serotonin production. Living in the country rather than the city is favorable, but is not likely to extend lifespan significantly beyond the average maximum. Although there are usually more negative ions in the country than in the city, positive ions still predominate five to four. This, again, is one of nature's little imperfections. The surface of our planet is negatively charged and therefore repels the highly mobile negative ions, forcing them to higher altitudes. Living in the mountains can offer a somewhat improved ion environment. Dwelling in the immediate vicinity of a waterfall could be even better. Plants and spray fountains in living areas can do much to remedy electrostatic conditions. We anticipate that in the near future, as the general populace becomes more aware of the ion phenomenon, negative-ion generators will be standard appliances in homes, offices, automobiles, and other spaces where human beings spend time.

There are four basic types of ionizer that are likely to be used commercially. Each of these mimics a natural method of ion generation. One uses ultraviolet light; the second uses high-voltage corona discharge, much like that of a lightning flash; the third employs radioactive beta particles; the fourth uses water spray. Except for ordinary fountains, the fourth device is not yet commercially available. If poorly designed, the first two may produce dangerous amounts of ozone, and the third may leak radioactive particles. If properly constructed, however, a negative-ion generator should present no side dangers, and is likely to give immediate improvements in health and feelings of well-being, not to mention the long-range possibilities of retarded aging and prolonged lifespan.

Even though it has been clearly demonstrated that improperly ionized air can lead to poor health and sometimes to premature death, there is no final evidence yet that negative ions will extend human or animal lifespan much beyond the average maximum. Most evidence, however, strongly suggests that atmospheric ions and other serotonin-control measures may help delay the release of pituitary blocking factors that appear to play roles in hastening aging. At the very least, we can be certain that a negatively charged atmosphere is generally beneficial to health, and this, in turn, may have some modest life-extension value. L-dopa or carbidopa may work synergistically with negative ions to enhance any life-prolonging capacities that they may have. If other life-extension measures, as described in this book, are also applied, the chances of enjoying phenomenal longevity are greatly increased.

# Chapter Nine

# Making Up for Lost Time

## Hormone Replacement

*Many hormones, including the sex steroids, dwindle as we age. The body also loses its ability to make full use of these substances. Hormone shots have made people look younger and feel better. They can also prevent heart attack. Other than that, they don't make us live longer than normal, but many scientists believe that if we can restore the body's ability to use the hormones and then give them in shots, we can extend human lifespan.*

Despite increasing evidence, it has not yet been proven that "death hormones" and "youth hormones" exist. Still, several significant changes in the endocrine system are known to take place in our bodies with age. The most poignantly evident of these changes occurs in the menopausal and postmenopausal female. Because of a sharp decline in estrogen production by the ovaries, immensely destructive changes take place in all parts of a woman's body. Cholesterol levels rise, muscle tone is lost, the skin becomes dry and thin, the vaginal tissues lose their moisture and suppleness, and the bones become demineralized, porous, and fragile. Much of the calcium that is robbed from the bones permeates the arterial walls and other tissues, depriving them of their elasticity. These changes are accompanied by numerous unpleasant symptoms, including irritability, hot flashes, night sweats, leg cramps, and depression.

Some men go through a similar climacteric, known as andropause, but the symptoms and physical changes are not nearly as severe as those of the female. Although the amount of testosterone (the main male hormone) in the blood decreases in older men, the decline is very gradual and the percentage of the drop is usually quite insignificant.[175] Still, there is generally a reduction in urinary excretion of 17-ketosteroids (testosterone and related hormones belong to this group) and a rise in follicle-stimulating hormone (FSH). This seems to imply that there are appreciable losses of some male hormones during senescence. [12]

Some of the known hormones can alter the aging rate and prevent degeneration of the liver, heart, kidneys, and skeletal muscle, but the decline of these hormones does not appear to be a primary cause of aging. Studies in the mid-1960s by Friedman and Friedman showed that whole extract of pituitary substances can measurably increase animal lifespan. [110] They also undertook to find out which of the many hormones of the posterior lobe were responsible for the effect. Both aldosterone and vasopressin, when given alone, showed signs of toxicity; but when combined, they demonstrated some beneficial influences. [111] A later study by Bodanszky and Engel indicated that another pituitary component, oxytocin, may inhibit aging. [26]

Several of the corticosteroids also have some antiaging properties. Hydrocortisone lengthens the postmitotic lifespan of human amniotic cells, stimulates some biochemical processes, and improves work performance. Unfortunately, it also lowers the immunologic defenses. This could have the advantage of decreasing the self-destructive autoimmune response, but is very likely to leave one prone to infection.

Corticosteroids in general are growth inhibitors. This fact led one researcher, D. Bellamy, to conjecture that lifespan could be extended by retarding development with these substances. In 1968, he added small amounts of prednisolone phosphate to the drinking water of a short-lived mouse strain, commencing after weaning and continuing throughout life. This resulted in a definite increase in lifespan over the controls, especially in the males. Several typical aging changes—collagen accumulation, increased calcium-to-collagen ratio, and liver nucleic-acid decline—were less pronounced in the treated animals. Since the inherently short life of this breed of mouse apparently results from a genetic autoimmune defect, the life extension caused by the hormone may have resulted from its immunosuppressive traits. [13] Another researcher has proposed that the corticosteroids may also stimulate RNA synthesis and counteract the RNA-inhibiting effects of age-accumulated histones. [205] It has been reported that corticosteroids, in general, can act upon chromosomes to alter the nature and timing of gene transcription. [310]

For human embryonic lung-fibroblast cells, the Hayflick Limit is fifty doublings, plus or minus ten. When cortisone is added to the tissue culture, there is an increase of about fifteen doublings. [52, 175, 219, 411, 412] There may be a number of reasons for this extension: DNA/RNA stimulation may be one; also the fact that corticosteroids stabilize lysosome membranes and prevent toxic leakage from these scavenger bodies. [175, 397, 398]

Another pituitary hormone, known as somatotrophin (STH) or growth hormone (GH), has experimentally prevented some of the outward signs of aging. When increasing amounts of the hormone were given to rats over a period of time, the larger dosages (up to 15 mg daily) prevented senile weight loss and gave the animals a more youthful appearance. But it did not extend lifespan or alter the pattern of decline to death. [95]

GH is an anabolic agent; that is, it promotes the retention of nitrogen for tissue building. Nitrogen retention also maintains the water and fat in the tissues at more typically youthful proportions. At the moment, the main problem with GH is the difficulty in obtaining it. Cattle and hog pituitaries have been the major source of GH used in rat experiments. Growth hormones from different animals have slightly different molecular structures. After a period of treatment, rat tissues become resistant to its beneficial effects, just as human diabetics may eventually develop immunity to the effectiveness of bovine insulin. Most animal GH has no effectiveness in humans, and it would take about a thousand human pituitaries to yield a daily dosage of 1,000 mg. [296]

In 1971, Choh Hao Li, director of the Hormone Research Laboratory in Berkeley, synthesized the human growth hormone (HGH) fairly accurately, but this man-made molecule has only 10 per cent of the activity of the natural hormone. [208, 402] Two other approaches to increasing HGH levels in aging people have been considered. One is to extract the natural hormone from large-scale tissue cultures of human pituitary cells. The other is to reactivate the production of HGH in the pituitary, either by electric stimulation of the hypothalamic/pituitary axis or by injections of human chorionic gonadotrophin (HCGH).

The fact that senile osteoporosis is a direct result of decreased estrogen production suggested replacement of the hormone as therapy for menopausal and postmenopausal women. [216, 229, 395] Estrogen replacement in conjunction with adequate exercise and nutrition, including ample calcium and vitamin D, has now been tried on many women and has prevented the loss of bone minerals. As might be expected, it also prevents or minimizes other menopause symptoms and confers a more youthful appearance to older women. [399]

Female hormones (estrogens) occur in both sexes, as do male hormones (androgens). Both the estrogens and the androgens are anabolic agents, and are useful in treating geriatric patients troubled with senile weight loss. Their use often results in improved appearance, increased physical strength, and reduced tissue calcification.

In 1967, the research team of Asdell, Doornenbal, Joshi, and Sperling tested the effects of estradiol benzoate implantations in castrated rats of both sexes. The hormone extended the lifespan of the males, but not that of the females. Similar experiments substituting the male hormone testosterone propionate shortened both male and female lifespan. [3]

Estradiol may tend to extend life because it stimulates the production of new collagen, which normally decreases with age because of cross-linkage.[141, 172] The life-shortening effect of testosterone could be attributed to the fact that large dosages of the hormone can cause lysosome leakage.[397] The combination of castration with testosterone implantation may also have had some bearing on the lifespan decrease.

Despite these findings, testosterone does have several positive influences on aging subjects, especially when a definite deficiency exists. It can improve vigor and muscle tone, and relieve nervous irritability and some aspects of mental senility in postandropausal men. It has been used effectively in various combinations with female steroids, such as estradiol benzoate, ethynylestradiol, and progesterone, to achieve both physiological and psychological benefits in geriatric patients.[19, 36]

Another life-preserving property of the estrogens is that they prevent cholesterol accumulation and the fatty degeneration of the arterial walls. For this reason, heart attack in premenopausal women is far less frequent than in males of the same age. In postmenopausal females, however, the coronary statistics more closely resemble those of males.[295]

There has been some concern over the use of male and female hormones, because they seem to promote tumors in mice and can produce opposite sex characteristics. But if they are administered properly and balanced when necessary with other steroids, the risk is minimized.[170] Estrogens have, in fact, been used with considerable success to treat prostatic carcinoma and some other cancers.

The endocrine system is amazingly complex. The effects of any one hormone in the body will depend largely on its proportional relationship to a welter of other hormones. Age, too, can make a vast difference in hormone responses. Some reactions in older animals are directly opposite to those in younger ones. Both hydrocortisone and vasopressin, for example, increase water loss in young rats, but decrease it in old ones.[12] There is also a loss of target sensitivity that often occurs in older animals; that is, the hormones may still be produced in adequate amounts, but the tissues that they are supposed to affect can no longer take them up or respond to them.[318] Furthermore, many hormonal reactions are due to the stimulation and activation of certain enzymes. Enzymes are complex protein molecules, built on RNA templates derived from DNA. Many of them contain, as part of their structures, specific metallic ions, such as zinc, manganese, selenium, or molybdenum. If faulty DNA/RNA results in missynthesized enzymes, or if mineral deficiencies lead to ion substitution, say, of copper for zinc, the hormone-induced chain of events will be altered, and the outcome will not be the same. Also, the hormones themselves may become altered as a result of protein error.

Frequently, a gland which has been overstimulated for a long period of time will simply become exhausted and cease to turn out its hormonal quota. Often, however, the diminution or

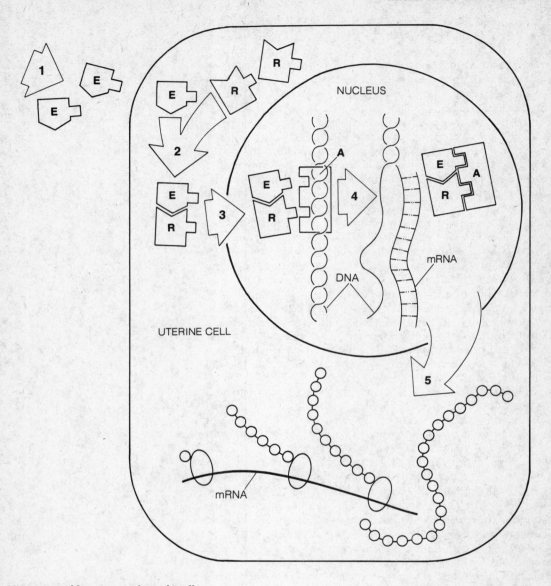

*How a steroid hormone works in the cell.*

The mechanism shown here has been found to be true for many hormones; here estrogen is used as an example. The hormone (E) circulates in the bloodstream, but concentrates in certain target cells, here the uterine cell. A special protein called a receptor (R) binds the estrogen molecule in a lock-and-key fashion. This complex moves into the nucleus, and by matching with a specific acceptor protein (A) associated with the "estrogen genes" causes that part of the DNA to be copied to mRNA. The mRNA then moves to the cytoplasm for translation to protein, and the cellular changes characteristic of estrogen response start. The role of the hormone, then, is to act directly to switch on a special DNA-to-mRNA transcription.

cessation of glandular function is caused not by any degeneration of the gland itself, but by a signal from the brain or nervous system. State of mind is profoundly related to glandular health. A happy, tranquil mind is likely to support healthy endocrines. Optimal hormonal secretions, in turn, engender a sound neural and mental state. Stress, on the other hand, may throw the endocrinal balances awry. The hypothalamus influences the pituitary to influence other glands. The hypothalamus itself can be influenced by such factors as general health, dietary and exercise

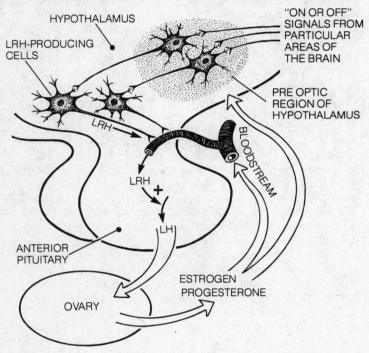

*How the brain regulates the amounts of estrogen and progesterone in the bloodstream and tissues.*

In this diagram, estrogen and progesterone are used as examples to show a process generally true for hormones. The cells in the preoptic region of the hypothalamus collect information from other regions of the brain and act as "timers" or cycle regulators. When activated, these nerve cells stimulate cells that produce LRH (luteinizing hormone-releasing hormone), which is secreted into the blood that enters the pituitary gland. In the pituitary, the LRH activates the production of LH (luteinizing hormone), which goes by the bloodstream to the ovary, where it turns on production of estrogen and progesterone. Estrogen and progesterone then act at specific target organs (uterine cells) and on the brain. In the brain, these steroids affect the system which started their synthesis and regions that influence sexual behavior. This chain of events shows one route by which the mental state is translated into hormone chemistry.

habits, brain and nerve conditions, atmospheric ionization, and serotonin levels. There is now considerable evidence that menopause is caused not by any failure in the ability of the ovaries to produce estrogen, but by a signal from the hypothalamic/pituitary axis that directs the ovaries to stop hormone manufacture and ovulation. Joseph Meites at Michigan State University has caused postmenopausal rats to resume estrogen production and ovulation by electrically stimulating particular centers of the brain, and by increasing brain levels of dopamine and norepinephrine.[309]

Hormone replacement therapy can be of undisputed value if certain steroids are in short supply because of age or illness. The anabolic nature of the steroids can assist tissue building in people who are run-down from these or other causes. Estrogen supplements will probably become standard therapy to reverse the wretched prank that nature plays on women of menopausal age.

Hormonal therapy is most effective when all other factors contributing to health and youth preservation are in order; e.g., diet, mental and neural health, adequate exercise, proper rest, and sufficient exposure to sunlight. The latter stimulates the endocrines through the eyes and skin surface. Antioxidants, such as vitamin E, prevent the destruction of the lipid portions of hormones in the tissues. Many people who appear to have hormone deficiencies are probably producing enough of the hormone, but much of it is oxidized before it can serve its purpose. With or without hormone replacement, many of the life-extension therapies described in this book can do much to preserve the normal endocrine function and prevent its decline.

Some synthetic anabolic steroids are now available by prescription. Among these are diethylstilbesterol, a synthetic type of estrogen used to promote cattle growth and as a morning-after contraceptive; and methandrostenolone, an artificial androgen that some body builders take when bucking to win a contest. These substances are not always reliable, and tend to produce many unwanted side effects. Long-term use of methandrostenolone can cause the gonads to decrease normal androgen production.[291] Such pseudohormones should be used for only brief periods, if used at all. Hormone-replacement therapy should be given only with natural steroids or exact synthetic replicas of these. Self-administration should never be attempted. Such therapy should not even be conducted by an ordinarily good physician, but rather by a competent endocrinologist with the best modern monitoring facilities available.

# Chapter Ten

# Romanian Rejuvenation

## *Gerovital H3*

*For several years, hundreds of thousands of people have flocked to Romania annually to get their shots of GH3, the controversial "youth drug" developed by Dr. Ana Aslan of Bucharest. Until recently, the drug was not permitted in the United States. Now the state of Nevada is allowing GH3 therapy. But people are still asking, "Does it really work? And what exactly is it supposed to do?"*

It has often been said that if our bodies could maintain homeostasis indefinitely, we might be immortal. Homeostasis is the chemical equilibrium of the body. The hypothalamus is very much involved in this aspect of biochemistry. Homeostasis regulates internal body temperature, blood pressure, perspiration rate, heart-pulse rate, blood sugar, hunger, thirst, sleeping and waking cycles, and almost every activity within the physical system. It also preserves the delicate balance between various enzymes, amines, and hormones in the body. As we age, many facets of our homeostatic harmony become imbalanced; unless they are compensated for, these imbalances may lead to far-reaching complications.

One aspect of homeostasis that alters with age and has a definite effect on some conditions of aging is the increase in monoamine oxidase (MAO) in the tissues. MAO is an enzyme that breaks down various amines that are formed in the body. Some of these amines, tyramine, for instance, are by-products of certain foods. Others are biogenic substances that occur naturally in the body and serve specific functions, such as aiding brain and nerve-impulse transmission. When, for example, the body produces extra epinephrine (adrenaline) or norepinephrine for added stimulation or emergency, MAO rapidly deaminates the excessive amounts of these neurohormones in the tissues and returns the body to its normal homeostatic balance.

Because MAO levels tend to rise with age, usually starting at around 45, greater than normal amounts of these stimulant amines are destroyed. When norepinephrine levels fall too low, activity of the brain and central nervous system is depressed. The anxiety, depression, and loss of interest in life that often accompany old age are now understood to be caused by excessive MAO, which causes a lack of norepinephrine and other catecholamines, especially in the hindbrain.[305] To correct this problem, physicians have usually prescribed MAO inhibitors or tricyclic compounds, which inactivate MAO. These drugs prevent the deamination of catecholamines in the brain and neuron vesicles, so that they can accumulate at the required levels. Depression is usually lifted, and energy increases enough that the person can function normally again.

Unfortunately, these MAO inhibitors have several disadvantages. The patient must avoid alcohol, amphetamines, and foods that are rich in tyramine or tyrosine (beer, chianti-type wines, and ripe cheeses), since these can interact with MAO inhibitors to cause a hypotensive crisis, which involves a sharp blood-pressure drop, chills, shivers, rapid heart palpitations, and breathing difficulties. Some combinations, though, can have an opposite effect, causing a steep blood-pressure rise (hypertensive crisis). Another disadvanatage of most MAO inhibitors is that their effects are not easily reversed. When the body needs more MAO to cope with toxins or infection, the inhibitor occupying the normal MAO sites decreases the activity of the enzyme.[180, 218]

How much excesses of MAO have to do with the aging process is still under investigation. The condition may be more a symptom than a cause of senescence. There is no question, however, that it is involved in most of the depression and anxiety that occur in later years. Depression and anxiety are forms of stress, and must inevitably have a deleterious effect on the body and accelerate aging. Mental attitude has been shown to reverberate on the endocrine systems, which in turn determine much of the body's total condition.

For many years, scientists and physicians have been looking for safer ways to control MAO levels in depressed or aging patients. Yet it appears that they may already have the agent they seek. It has been on every physician's shelf for the past sixty years. That substance is procaine, better known as novacaine.

## Procaine and Ana Aslan

Procaine was first synthesized by Alfred Einhorn in 1905. It was developed primarily as a local anesthetic to substitute for cocaine, which had turned out to have unmanageable side effects. In

1940, F. J. Philpot reported in the *Journal of Physiology* his discovery that procaine was, at least *in vitro*, an MAO inhibitor.[290] Nothing came of his finding at the time. A few enlightened physicians had noted that procaine injections relieved some forms of arthritis, but it was never established as a standard medication for this disorder.

Ana Aslan was born in Bucharest in 1899. She earned her medical degree in 1924 and became Romania's first female physician as well as its first cardiologist. During the late 1940s, as director of the government clinic at Timisoara in Romania, Dr. Aslan began using procaine injections to treat arthritis, angina pectoris, and other painful disorders. She had remarkable success in achieving the expected results, but what intrigued Aslan and her co-workers were the unexpected results, which could not be attributed to its local-anesthetic properties. Among other things, older patients felt younger and more alive, less depressed and more energetic.

In 1951, Dr. Aslan became director of the Bucharest Geriatric Institute, and developed an improved procaine compound, which she called Gerovital H3 or GH3. Her GH3 formula consists of 200 mg of procaine hydrochloride in 10 ml of saline solution, with 16 mg of benzoic acid and 14 mg of potassium metabisulfite, buffered to a slightly acid pH of 3.3.[218] It is usually administered intramuscularly three times a week for four weeks. This is followed by a rest period of two to four weeks, after which another series of injections or tablets is given. With this drug she observed many other antiaging effects: high cholesterol levels dropped; skin elasticity improved; skin texture became smoother and less wrinkled; muscular strength increased; hair often regrew on balding areas; pigmentation was sometimes restored to graying hair; high and low blood pressure were normalized; and even failing memory was greatly improved.

In 1956, Ana Aslan reported her findings at a symposium in Karlsruhe, West Germany.[4] Her claims were met largely with disbelief. The following year, supported by further evidence, she addressed another symposium, and this time was well-received. Soon other researchers were corroborating her findings. Studies in France and Germany showed a 20 to 30 per cent increase in the lifespan of rats given regular injections of GH3.

In the early 1960s, however, some British and American workers challenged Aslan's discoveries. They had attempted to duplicate her experiments, using ordinary procaine hydrochloride instead of her GH3 preparation, and quite understandably did not get the same results.[16, 98, 117, 143, 221] The AMA, brandishing all negative findings and ignoring all positive ones, officially declared GH3 (procaine) useless as anything other than a local anesthetic.[388] Despite the fact that the AMA is notorious for its blatantly unscientific habit of arriving at conclusions that suit

*Procaine*
Procaine is the main ingredient of Gerovital.

its own prejudices and purposes, the statement was enough to dampen American interest in GH3 for ten years.

The destiny of this drug took a new turn in 1965, when a research group at the Chicago Medical School headed by Arnold Abrams published the results of a series of carefully controlled double-blind tests with both GH3 and ordinary procaine. The intent of the experiments had been to disprove the claims made for the Romanian drug, but the honest conclusion these workers had to report was that, although procaine yielded only slight results, GH3 had beneficial physical and psychological effects that warranted further study. [1]

In 1971, Alfred Sapse of UCLA revived interest in GH3 in the United States. He ran a computer check on all available procaine data, and received readouts that completely supported the idea that the drug is efficacious. He then had M. David MacFarlane of the University of Southern California test GH3 as an MAO inhibitor. MacFarlane reported that it is a mild, short-acting, selective, fully competitive, and reversible MAO inhibitor. [217] That is, GH3 inhibits certain forms of MAO that are effective in neutralizing particular catecholamines, such as nor-epinephrine and serotonin, but has very little effect on others. It competes for MAO sites, but does not cling to them permanently. If extra MAO is needed, the inhibitor is easily displaced. Another advantage of GH3 as an MAO inhibitor is that the patient does not have to shun alcohol and certain foods and drugs in order to avoid hypotensive and hypertensive crises. [321]

After Sapse was thoroughly convinced of GH3's value as an MAO inhibitor and antiaging drug, he joined forces with Manfred Mosk and Nathan Kline and founded Rom-American Pharmaceuticals, Ltd. They negotiated with the Romanian government, and won a ten-year contract for exclusive rights to import the drug into the United States and to distribute it. Seven years later, Rom-Amer was still trying to gain FDA approval merely to conduct clinical tests with GH3 in this country. Finally, the company had to move from California to Nevada, the only state that no longer bans the drug. Since ordinary anesthetic procaine has been in common use for more than half a century, there is no serious question about its safety. Further information about its worth can only be derived by clinical testing. The main obstacle seems to be the FDA's general reluctance to approve foreign-produced drugs.

The public's interest in the reports of GH3's beneficial effects, coupled with the unavailability of the substance in this country, has created a market for inferior products that bear names similar to Gerovitol or GH3, but that contain no procaine. In Europe, however, several worthy variations on Dr. Aslan's formula are produced and sold. Doctors Wolfgang Schwartzhaupt and Fritz Wiedermann have developed an oral version of the drug, potentiated with hematoporphyrin, and known as KH3.

Hematoporphyrin has a regulating effect on the nervous system, is used for treating nervous depression, and also improves the functionings of the sexual glands. [193, 231]

Since excessive serotonin is known to be harmful and is now regarded as a probable trigger for the "death hormone" responses, it may seem contradictory that one of procaine's virtues is that it prevents the deamination of this and other catecholamines, thus allowing them to accumulate. There is no actual contradiction, however. Brain amines, such as serotonin, dopamine, and norepinephrine, exist in a balanced relationship with each other, varying somewhat in different sections of the brain. The limbic structures, for instance, contain the highest concentrations of serotonin and norepinephrine, whereas the neocortical portions have almost none. In most brain tissues, the distributions of these two neurohormones are more or less similar. The hypothalamus has less serotonin, but the proportion increases with age. The "death hormone" response appears to be triggered by an abnormal rise of serotonin and a simultaneous depletion of dopamine, the precursor of norepinephrine, in this organ. The object of using L-dopa and negative ions to control serotonin, then, is not to rid the brain tissues of this neurohormone, but rather to normalize its distribution in proportion to the other amines.

Although procaine is a synthetic chemical, it is composed of two natural substances: para-aminobenzoic acid (the B vitamin, PABA) and diethylaminoethanol (DEAE, which apparently participates in the synthesis of choline and acetylcholine;[6, 8, 123] it is similar to DMAE, which was discussed in Chapter 2). When procaine enters the bloodstream, it is rapidly hydrolyzed into these two substances. [173] For a while, some gerontologists believed that the benefits of procaine and GH3 might be entirely due to the vitamin effects of these two metabolites. But equivalent dosages of PABA and DEAE did not produce the same results as the drug. [6] It has been suggested that procaine may reach important sites in the brain or in the individual cells not ordinarily permeated by PABA or DEAE, and is then converted to these vitamins. [41]

Although the benzoic acid and potassium metabisulfite are added to GH3 as antioxidants and preservatives, they seem to have additional functions. The presence of the potassium ion aids in the absorption of the drug, and the benzoic acid may partially form a benzoate salt of procaine. This may slow down the otherwise rapid metabolism of the procaine and give it more time to accomplish its work. [8]

It is not well understood why GH3 is so much more effective than procaine. Its gentle MAO-inhibiting properties explain its value in treating anxiety, depression, and abnormal blood pressure, but it also has a stimulating influence on cells and tissues. The late J. Earl Officer at the USC School of Medicine administered GH3 to embryonic wild-mouse tissue cultures during maturation and again during the normal decline period. He found that the aging of the cells was slowed down and possibly reversed.[248] Ana Aslan had previously had similar results using chick- and monkey-cell cultures.[5]

B. M. Zuckerman at the University of Massachusetss Laboratory of Experimental Biology slowed the aging process in a species of nematode by adding GH3 to its medium. Many aging traits of this nematode are similar to those of human red blood cells. Both accumulate the aging pigment lipofuscin. Also, the cell membranes of both become fragile with age, while the cell becomes heavier and loses its negative surface charge. GH3 retards the formation of lipofuscin in nematodes, and inhibits the development of liver spots (lipofuscin deposits) in humans.[414] GH3 seems to strengthen cell membranes, according to studies now in progress.

GH3 may not be the key to extraordinary life extension, but it appears to help treat and delay the onset of many of the symptoms and side effects of aging. It can be a useful adjuvant to other longevity agents, and will, most likely, potentiate their effectiveness.

# Chapter Eleven
# Other Attacks on Aging

*In the preceding chapters, we have examined some of the more common measures being employed or considered by gerontologists and self-experimenting longevists for controlling or minimizing the effects of aging. These were emphasized either because there is a fair accumulation of knowledge about them, or because they directly affect some of the better known and established causes of aging. They are by no means the only approaches being practiced today. Several other avenues of attack on the aging disease deserve at least some mention, because of either their effectiveness or their popularity.*

## Cell Therapy

In April 1931, when a Swiss surgeon accidentally damaged the parathyroid glands of a woman in her sixties during a goiter operation, the brilliant surgeon Dr. Paul Niehans was called to try to save the woman's life. As a last resort, he prepared a physiological solution of the cellular material from the parathyroids of a freshly slaughtered steer and injected this into the dying woman's pectoral muscles. She showed signs of recovery almost immediately, and ultimately lived into her nineties.

This was the beginning of cell therapy, a technique that is now practiced at many clinics in Europe and elsewhere. It entails the injection of fresh, living cells from specific organs of a sheep fetus, taken one month before scheduled birth. Sheep are the preferred source because of their high resistance to disease. Organs that do not develop sufficiently in the fetus, such as testes, ovaries, adrenals, parathyroids, and the pituitary, are taken from a mature animal. The organs are diced, placed in 20 cc. of saline solution, and further chopped. The solution is then injected intramuscularly into the patient. No more than two hours, and

"The heart heals the heart, lung heals lung, spleen heals spleen; *similia similibus curantur* (like cures like)."

Paracelsus
(early sixteenth-century alchemist)

preferably only one hour, may elapse between slaughter and injection.

When a particular organ in the patient is functioning poorly, cells from the same organ of a sheep are injected. The young cells somehow impart to the failing organ the ability to function properly again. It does not seem to matter that the cells are from a foreign species; only that they are from the same organ. Even Paul Niehans was unable to explain how cell therapy works. One hypothesis is that the DNA and RNA of the donor cells transfer to the cells of the defective organ the genetic information required for them to function properly. Another explanation is that certain chemicals present in the injected cells may initiate a chain of events that stimulates the host to activate the failing system. However it works, cell therapy's positive influence on living organisms is so great that it cannot be used if there is serious infection in the patient, or else it may cause rampant proliferation of bacillary activity.

As a result of the improvements in all the organs being treated, cell therapy seems to have a rejuvenating effect on the entire body. Skin tone is so greatly improved that many European hospitals include cell therapy in the post-operative treatment after facelifts and other cosmetic surgery for the aging. Although fresh cells give the best results, some clinics use lyophilized (freeze-dried) or fresh-frozen cells.

Cell therapy has been performed successfully on tens of thousands of people, including many well-known actors, authors, artists, and politicians. In 1954, the ailing Pope Pius XII received cell therapy from Niehans after Vatican physicians had given a fatal prognosis. After his astonishing recovery, the Pope rewarded Niehans with a fellowship in the Pontifical Academy. The chair that Niehans occupied was the one left vacant upon the death of Sir Arthur Fleming, whose own discovery, penicillin, had been suppressed for many years by the gray faces of orthodox medicine. Despite its many successes, cell therapy is heavily criticized in most orthodox medical circles. In the United States, the FDA does not permit the practice of this technique, nor even the importation of freeze-dried cells.

In 1963 Dr. Alfred Kment, a Viennese veterinarian, studied the effects of cell therapy on aging animals. Endurance levels, tested on a rotating exercise drum, were greatly increased. This improvement lasted about ten days. Memory, learning, and intelligence, tested in a maze, were also improved. Healing was as rapid as in youth; connective tissues were characteristic of younger animals; and further cross-linkage of the tissues was inhibited. [181]

As mentioned in Chapter 7, foreign cells are usually rejected by the immunological system. Although the cells in Niehans' therapy are from a different animal—not just another human—they are apparently accepted. The rule here seems to be that if a system is failing and receives vital cells, they will be accepted and used for revitalization. If the system is functioning well, they will have no effect and will be harmlessly rejected. [244]

It has been considered that cell therapy could be more effective, though, if cells or RNA injected into an aging person were from his own younger body. Dr. John H. Heller, Executive Director of the New England Institute of Medical Research at Ridgefield, Connecticut, has proposed that cells, or nucleic acids from the cells, could be taken from a person during youth, frozen in liquid helium, and reinjected at various periods of life when degenerative changes begin to occur. At the time of this writing, this experiment has been successfully accomplished with tissue cultures, but not with humans or animals. [226] As reported in Chapter 7, Makinodan has succeeded in a similar experiment in which he rejuvenated the immune systems of aging animals by injecting them with frozen lymphocytes from their younger days.

## Sulfonamides

Several workers have reported that animals live longer and show signs of rejuvenation and improved health when they receive small daily doses of sulfa drugs, especially sulfadiazine. [125] Human geriatric patients have experienced improvements in hearing, vision, sexual function, tissue condition, and general health when treated with a combination of sulfadiazine, magnesium ascorbate, and calcium pantothenate. [303] The daily use of sulfadiazine would very likely produce a resistance to all sulfa drugs and render them useless as antibiotics. This may not be a serious problem, however, since they have been largely replaced by other drugs. Medical dosages of sulfadiazine range between 500 and 4,000 mg. About one patient out of a thousand has toxic side reactions to the drug, even though it is the least toxic of the sulfa group. I and several acquaintances have experimented with daily dosages of 250 mg of sulfadiazine plus 500 mg each of the ascorbate and the pantothenate. Satisfactory results were noted, and there were no toxic reactions. Sulfa drugs interfere with the B vitamin PABA, however; so it is important to obtain enough PABA when using a sulfa drug regularly as an aging control. The sulfonamides also tend to deplete intestinal flora, which should be well-supplemented, since they synthesize many of the body's B vitamins. To replace the flora, take liquid or freeze-dried acidophilus, which can be bought at health-food stores, and should contain a mixture of Lactobacillus Acidophilus, Bulgaricus, and Caucasicus. Flora require lactose for nourishment. If milk products are not included in the diet, a teaspoonful or more of milk sugar can be taken daily.

*Sulfadiazine*

## Fasting and Detoxification

For many years before life-extension drugs were available, thousands of longevity-seekers went on periodic fasts or detoxification diets to allow the body to rid itself of toxic waste products. The effectiveness of fasting as a life-extension measure is fairly well backed by experimental evidence. In one study, rats that were made to fast for one day out of three throughout life had a 20 per cent lifespan increase. This approach had nothing to do with McCay's calorie-restriction experiments, described in Chapter 8. Puberty was not delayed, and growth was not stunted. [292]

There are many books on fasting available at most health-food stores. Some advocate total fasts, during which only water is taken. Others recommend partial fasts, or mono-fasts, in which only a single nutriment—usually a fruit or vegetable juice—is consumed.

The general rules of fasting are simple, but important.

1. Be in reasonably good condition before you start the fast. Your body should be well-rested and not suffering from any nutritional deficiency.

2. Never begin a fast on a day when you have already eaten. Eat lightly the night before the fast. A bowl of yogurt or a glass or two of kefir is perfect, because these provide acidophilus bacteria, which aid in detoxification and the manufacture of many of the B vitamins.

3. During the fast, drink plenty of distilled or spring water (never drink tap water). This helps to allay hunger and flushes toxins from the tissues. A teaspoonful of ascorbic acid added to each quart of water aids in detoxification, but is weak enough not to cause an acid stomach.

4. The peristalsic movements of the lower intestine continue during fasting, so there are bowel movements, but there is no bulk or fiber to cleanse the lower tract and keep waste materials moving through. For this reason many experts recommend an enema on the first morning, and another at the end of the fast. Some people also take a dose of psyllium seeds each day of the fast. Taken with water, they expand in the stomach and provide bulk. They are completely indigestible and serve only as an aid to elimination. The seed hulls provide roughage, and the water and nonnutritive seed-oils give lubrication. They are available from herb dealers and drugstores. A powdered form is produced by Searle Laboratories under the brand name Metamucil.

5. Get plenty of rest, relaxation, fresh air, and sunlight while fasting. Some people experience a slight headache during the early part of a fast. This usually passes after a short while. Water, fresh air, and a tranquil mind help relieve it.

6. Don't exercise heavily during the fast. Light exercise, though, helps the tissues dispel toxic wastes.

7. Avoid mental, physical, and nervous stress.

8. Don't smoke marijuana during a fast if it tends to stimulate your appetite.

9. When breaking the fast, don't shock your body with food. Start with a nonacidic juice (apple, prune, grape, or vegetable, rather than citrus). This will reawaken your digestive system, and bring blood sugars up to normal. An hour or so later, have some yogurt, kefir, or buttermilk. These are easily digested, and increase intestinal flora. A few hours later, a light, solid meal can be taken. One or two soft-boiled, poached, or scrambled eggs is a good choice. After you digest this, you can return to normal eating habits. The longer the fast, the more gradual the reintroduction of food should be. Some people take multivitamins and chelated minerals during the fast, so that the body's reserves of these are not depleted.

10. If you are not used to fasting, your first fast should not exceed one day. If you wish eventually to fast for several days, build up to it gradually. [292]

## Stress Avoidance

Throughout this book, the dangers of stress have been reiterated. Perhaps this word "stress" requires some defining and qualifying. Anything that places demands on the body is stress. But demands on the body are inevitable, natural, and necessary for development and well-being. Exercise, for instance, is a form of stress, but, when it is properly applied, it makes the body stronger. Overexercise, on the other hand, tears the body down faster than it can rebuild itself. As surely as overexercise is stress, so is lack of exercise. The term stress, as used in this and most other writings, actually refers to overstress, that is, anything that places undue demands on the body, resulting in adverse reactions.

Stress is probably one of the major causes of premature aging and death. In a sense, we have been talking about stress in every chapter of this book. Toxins create stress, and stress creates toxins. So do infections, exhaustion, poorly ionized air, senile MAO increases, free radicals, nutritional deficiencies, and an improperly functioning immune system. Stress can cause increases in serotonin, and large amounts of serotonin can induce further stress. We have already seen how extreme stress can incite the overproduction of pituitary factors; these factors stimulate the adrenals to secrete excessive amounts of corticosteroids, which in turn distort the normal potassium-to-sodium balance in the cardiac muscles, resulting in heart attack.

Almost every antiaging measure we have covered in this book is also an antistress measure. Some, such as antistress vitamins and minerals, are by definition immediate attempts to cope with this destructive factor. Along with all the chemical and physical tools for stress reduction and life extension that have

"If we kept throughout life the same resistance to stress, injury, and disease that we had at the age of ten, about one half of us here today might expect to survive in seven hundred years' time."

Alex Comfort,
*Ageing: The Biology of Senescence*

been touched on in these chapters, mental attitude is of key importance. A perturbed mind augments stress throughout the body; a tranquil mind reduces stress. The possible paths toward peace of mind are legion. Relaxation approaches derived from yoga, Zen, tai chi, aikido, transcendental meditation, biofeed-back, primal therapy, Jacobsen relaxation technique, etc., all have something valid to offer. [168] You will need to find what works best for you. [333]

## Herbs and Longevity

No book on life extension would be complete without some mention of the venerable herbalist Li Chung Yun, who, according to Chinese government records, was born in 1677 and died in 1933 at the age of 256. He supposedly appeared to be about 50 when he was 200, and was living with his twenty-fourth wife at the time of his death. He attributed his longevity to strict vege-tarianism, correct walking, breathing, and sleeping habits, and the daily use of ginseng and another herbal material called *fo-ti-tieng*. In *Nature's Medicine*, Richard Lucas translates *fo-ti-tieng* as "elixir of long life," and states that it is the Asian marsh penny-wort (*Hydrocotyle asiatica minor*). Lucas reports that the French biochemist Jules Lepin and Professor Ménier of the Académie Scientifique discovered a substance in the plant that has a rejuve-nating effect on the nerves, brain, and endocrines. Lucas also writes about another plant called *gotu kola* (*Centella asiatica*), which has similar properties, and which people in Ceylon and southern Asia take to retain youth and promote longevity. [214] In fact, the *Hydrocotyle* and *Centella* plants are merely geographical variants of the same species, the latter sometimes growing slightly larger than the former. [122]

There has also been some debate over the actual identity of Li's *fo-ti-tieng* elixir. Dr. Leung Kok Yuen of the North American College of Acupuncture believes that it was not the Asian penny-wort, but the tuber of the fleeceflower plant (*Polygonum multi-flori*). This herb is reputed to strengthen bone, blood, muscle, and internal organs. [122]

The greatest controversy, naturally, concerns Li's true age. Some critics insist that there were two Li Chung Yuns: the father, born in 1677; and the son, who died in 1933. If these skeptics are correct, one may still be impressed by these two men, each of whom must have lived about 150 years.

Many modern herbalists and longevists swear by *gotu kola* as a brain stimulant, detoxifying agent, and cell energizer, but there has been little if any serious scientific study of its chemistry and pharmacology. Ginseng (*Panax ginseng*), however, has received some attention from scientists. Studies have revealed that sub-stances in this herbal root increase mental efficiency, prevent fatigue, purify the blood, protect against radiation, hinder cell degeneration in postmitotic cells, increase resistance to stress and infection, reduce accumulation of cholesterol by improving its metabolism, improve the synthesis of RNA and protein in the liver, and stimulate circulation, digestion, endocrine activity, and general metabolism.[112, 251, 322, 390] Soviet scientists have found that some of these substances are also antioxidants and free-radical deactivators.[390] Harman has reported that the lifespan of fruit flies has been experimentally extended with ginseng. Two other related plants, Siberian ginseng (*Eleutherococcus senticosus*) and American ginseng (*Panax quinquefolius*), possess properties similar to those of the Chinese species.[30]

A small piece of ginseng root can be chewed, or a tea can be made by adding hot water to a slurry of the powdered root. A tea can also be made by steeping one or two heaping teaspoonfuls of *gotu kola* leaves in a cup of boiled water. The rock-hard tubers of the fleeceflower plant must be boiled for six hours in two quarts of water, adding water as needed to maintain volume. One-half to one pint of this is taken daily.

# Chapter Twelve
# Starting the Life-
# Extension Program

Life may be viewed as a series of episodes that function as a failsafe system to ensure our individual deaths. If one thing doesn't kill us, another surely will. More than likely, though, all our internal self-destruct mechanisms will collaborate to bring about the gradual but thorough devastation of our bodies. Perhaps gerontologists will one day discover a single, pivotal cause of all aging conditions and a drug that will counteract it. For now, however, the best we can do is regard the known causes of aging as a group of assailants, each attacking a different system in the body with its own weapon, and each weakening the body's protections in its own way, so that the entire organism becomes more vulnerable to all assaults. As we are attacked on all fronts at once, so we must resist on all fronts, while bearing in mind that a fortress is only as strong as its weakest wall of defense. Our eventual defeat by this collective enemy must be accepted as inevitable. All that the longevist can really hope for is to hold out against this enemy for as long as possible, and to derive as much enjoyment and fulfillment as he can from whatever time is gained.

Although we do not yet know what prevents us from living to be 200, we do have a good body of information about what keeps us from reaching 120. We also have a number of therapies that are expected to overcome this limitation. Throughout this book I have tried to make absolutely clear the degrees of certainty and uncertainty about the probable effectiveness of these therapies in humans. The intent of this book has been to describe the current state of knowledge in gerontology, and to examine various agents that offer some protection against the causes and symptoms of aging. Since many people are already using or planning to use some of these treatments, I have tried to supply information that will help them do so sensibly. I am not saying, "Take these therapies and drugs, and you will feel better and live longer." I am saying, "People I know and trust have been experimenting on themselves with these agents, and have learned a few things about them though experience, lectures, literature, and personal conversations with leading gerontologists." I do not urge you to commence a life-extension program, but if you are going to commence one, I hope you will first become familiar with the material in this book.

## Longevity and the Mind

Many scientists and writers have said that after the age of 35, there is a daily loss of about 10,000 irreplaceable neural cells in the brain, and that a very old person has approximately half the number of functioning brain cells that he had as a young adult. This rate of loss is now seriously doubted by most researchers.[183, 386] Although we may suffer great depletions when we abuse ourselves with alcohol, nicotine, or other drugs, or suffer from other extraordinary stresses, the rate of brain-cell death is not consistently this high. If the loss of 10,000 a day were continuous from age 35, the successful longevist, on this three-hundredth birthday, would have a zero population of active brain neurons. What a horrid joke this would be on gerontology's crowning achievement! A magnificent specimen, three centuries young, looking gorgeous, and bursting with vigor, but a drooling idiot!

It is improbable, however, that this is the actual fate of the longevist. Although there are permanent losses of neuronal cells throughout life, these do not necessarily lead to mental incompetence. Even when large masses of brain tissue are destroyed or removed, the remaining cells can take over their functions, and the loss may be scarcely noticed. Nevertheless, there is often a reduction of mental capacity and intellectual energy in the aged. Rather than being the result of decreased numbers of brain cells, senile dementia appears to be due to changes in and around these cells. These changes may include senile plaque formation from amyloidosis, decline of RNA synthesis, toxic metal accumulations,[282] impaired oxidative metabolism, reduced circulation, damaged or hardened blood vessels in the brain, and the diminishing of certain catecholamines and their receptor sites. Lipid peroxidation in cell membranes, cross-linkage of brain tissue, and lipofuscin accumulation may also contribute to mental decline during aging.

Throughout this book, we have considered the effects of these aging factors on the cells of both the body in general and the brain. Most of the antiaging therapies that we have discussed can be expected to contribute as much toward the preservation of the brain as toward that of any other organ of the body; so there is no need to make an in-depth study of the problems of brain senescence. It may be of interest, though, to take a cursory glance at some of the new drugs that show promise in coping directly with mental senility.

## Mind

Some scientists, like Lawrence Casler, SUNY/Geneseo psychologist, have been experimenting with hypnosis and life extension. Casler has implanted posthypnotic suggestions for longevity in volunteer students, and they have agreed to stay in lifelong contact with him. The experiment, of course, will take a century or more to complete. Casler has also tried this on older people; so we may have some reports in 20 or 30 years.

**Typical vitamins and minerals that a well-informed longevist might use as part of a life-extension program.**

| NAME | DOSAGE RANGE | TO BE TAKEN |
|---|---|---|
| Vitamin A | 20,000–30,000 I.U. | divided, with meals |
| Vit. D | 3,000–5,000 I.U. | same |
| Vit. E | 800–1,200 I.U. | same |
| Vit. C | 5,000–15,000 mg | between meals, in liquids |
| Vit. B1 | 25–100 mg (200–1,000 mg under stress) | divided, with meals or between |
| Vit. B2 | 50–100 mg (200–300 mg under stress) | same |
| Vit. B3, niacin(amide) | 200–500 mg (up to 3,000 mg under stress) | same |
| Vit. B5, pantothenate | 100–1,200 mg | same |
| Vit. B6, pyrodoxine | 50–100 mg (500 mg under stress) | same |
| PABA | 500–1,000 mg (3,000 mg under stress or ozone) | same |
| Choline | 1,000–3,000 mg | same |
| Inositol | 1,000–3,000 mg | same |
| Folic acid | 5 mg (or 1 mg per 300 mg of B5) | same |
| Biotin | 100 mcg per 300 mg of B5 | same |
| Vit. B12 | 25 mcg (500–3,000 mcg by injection each 3–7 days) | same |
| Vit. B15, pangamate | 150–250 mg | same |
| Nucleic acids | 1,000–2,000 mg | dietetically (see Table 1) or supplementally with meals |
| Rutin – bioflavonoid | 100 mg (200–400 mg at times) | with meals or blender drinks |
| Calcium | 1,000–1,600 mg | divided, with acid fruit or juice |
| Magnesium | 500–800 mg | same |
| Zinc | 40–70 mg | divided, with meals |
| Manganese | 15–25 mg | with meals |
| Chromium | 250–1,000 mcg | no supplement needed if 2 Tbs. of brewer's yeast is taken |
| Molybdenum | 500–1,000 mcg | divided, with meals |
| Sulfur (flowers) | 200–400 mg | with yogurt, kefir, or acidophilus |
| Methionine HCl | 500–1,000 mg | divided, with meals |
| Cysteine HCl | 500–2,000 mg | same |
| Deanol | 100–400 mg | in morning |
| Ascorbyl palmitate | 1,000–2,000 mg | added to foods |
| 2-MEA | 100–200 mg | divided, with meals |
| L-dopa | 1,000–3,000 mg | same |
| Thiodipropionic acid | 200 mg | added to foods or in hot water |
| BHA or BHT | 200 mg | dissolved in oils |

## Typical Vitamins and Minerals *continued*

| | | |
|---|---|---|
| Ethoxyquin | 50–100 mg | same |
| Sulfadiazine | 100–250 mg | anytime |
| GH3, procaine | 200 mg | as administered or prescribed by clinic or physician |
| Ginseng | 1–3 grams | chewed or in tea |
| Gotu kola | 1–2 cups of tea and/or 5–20 fresh leaves | taken early in day if stimulating |
| Fleeceflower infusion | ½–1 pint | prepared as described in text |

Hydergine (dihydroergotoxine) is a nonhallucinogenic lysergic-acid derivative produced by Sandoz Pharmaceuticals. When administered for a period of time, it accumulates in specific areas of the brain, especially in the synapses and the pituitary.[167] In these places, it acts on energy metabolism and improves the utilization of oxygen.[39, 92] It also regulates the metabolism of cyclic-AMP,[93] which is sometimes called the "second messenger." When a hormone (the first messenger) becomes bound to the receptor site of its target-cell membrane, cyclic-AMP is produced, and delivers the hormonal message within the cell.[305, 375] Hydergine also facilitates the synthesis of brain protein and normalizes EEG responses.[39, 92]

PMH (pemoline magnesium hydroxide) manufactured by Abbott Laboratories under the brand name Cylert, acts as an antidepressant and mild central-nervous-system stimulant, but has no addictive potential or harmful side effects. Some workers have reported that it improves learning and memory, and increases RNA synthesis in the brain;[118, 293, 344] however, most researchers have not been able to duplicate these results.[28, 91, 236, 356] PMH's influence on learning and remembering may be due to its general alerting effect. More study of it is needed.

Ribamol (2-hydroxytriethylammonium ribonucleate), another drug that is under investigation, is also said to enhance memory and learning.[59]

Methisprinol, also called isoprinosine, has been found by Paul Gordon to partially reverse deterioration of brain function in rats. Among other things, it increases RNA synthesis in brain cells. It is chemically related to DMAE.[315]

Piracetem (Nootropyl) is a new drug that appears to improve verbal memory, but not other kinds of memory, according to S. J. Dimond and E. Y. M. Brouwers of the University College in Cardiff, Wales.[209]

Vincamine is an alkaloid found in the leaves of the Madagascar periwinkle (*Catharanthus roseus*, formerly *Vinca Rosea*). Alkaloids from this plant have some reputation as anticancer agents. Vincamine has also proven somewhat useful in combatting mental decline caused by cerebrovascular disorders.[315] Vinca alkaloids, however, can have many undesirable side effects, including white-corpuscle reduction and muscle-tissue degeneration. [54, 291]

Several other drugs, such as strychnine sulfate, picrotoxine, diazadamantol, bemegride, and pentylenetetrazol (Metrazol), administered in doses well below the convulsive threshold, can facilitate learning and may be of some value in treating senility problems. [224]

Carl C. Pfeiffer and others have linked senility to low blood-spermine levels. Spermine is a simple polyamine that is found in the blood, brain, and semen. The synthesis of RNA in the brain, which is essential for recent-memory retention, requires RNA polymerase, which is activated by spermine. Tests conducted at the Brain Bio Center at Princeton showed spermine concentrations to be low in senile and presenile patients who had poor memories for recent events, but high in those with adequate memories. Spermine levels are known to decline during aging, and in persons with hypoglycemia or on estrogen therapy. Pfeiffer claims that supplementation of trace minerals, especially manganese and zinc, can raise spermine levels and relieve mental confusion and memory loss in the aged. [279]

It has been suggested that preventing declines in brain function may positively influence the longevity of the body. The cybernetic aging theory of J. W. Still holds that aging is partly caused by a decline in message transmission in the neuroendocrine system, which is caused in turn by a loss of functional brain cells. [360] The fact that children with Downes' syndrome (Mongolism) or severe brain damage display premature aging signs and die at an early age lends some support to this theory. [90] Whether Still is correct or not, it is generally agreed that an active mind and healthy mental attitude is of paramount importance for the longevity and well-being of the aged.

There has been much recent interest in intelligence-boosting drugs. These can help the elderly to regain lost brain function, but are also of value to younger people who want to increase their brainpower or get better mileage from their minds. An excellent article by Sandy Shakocius and Durk Pearson in *Omni* (May 1979) described many of these drugs and their use, and included a list of references. I recommend this article to anyone wishing to explore the subject.

## Life-Extension Drugs and the Law

A few of the life-extension drugs described in this book can be obtained only by prescription, but most are freely available from the suppliers listed in Appendix A. A major reason why so few of these substances are controlled by government agencies is that so few people know about them. This fortunate situation may change after the publication of this book.

Before the psychedelic movement of the middle and late 1960s, many psychoactive agents were readily obtainable from legitimate chemical companies. Unlike marijuana, cocaine, and other "street drugs" of minority cultures, exotic substances such as ibogaine, psilocybin, and dimethyltryptamine had not, in the eyes of the authorities, presented any social problem. Virtually no one had even heard of them. In October 1970, under Title 21 of the United States Code, many of these "unheard-of" substances became illicit.

Mind drugs, though, are not the only materials that the federal government has declared war on. The FDA has been trying for years to control the sales of ordinary vitamins, and to limit the allowable dosages of pills to almost useless amounts. Most of their attempts in this direction have been defeated so far. Nevertheless, they have had some victories. Laetrile, the controversial anticancer agent, is found in many foods and has vitamin-like properties. Yet it is illegal in its pure form. Vitamin $B_{15}$ (pangamic acid), though not federally controlled, is forbidden in many states. We have already discussed the legal status of GH3 in this country.

The question that concerns most longevists is, what do we do when the FDA forbids the sale of life-extension drugs? After this happens, there may be little we can do, but by acting beforehand, we may be able to prevent such a catastrophe.

According to the judicial interpretation of the First Amendment of the Constitution of the United States, no government agency can interfere with a person's right to use a religious sacrament, unless that substance was already illegal at the time it was declared to be a sacrament. It would now be impossible, for example, for a church to declare cocaine, marijuana, LSD, or any other illegal material to be a sacrament. But if a substance were already believed to be a sacrament before it was declared illegal, its availability to church members could not be denied. For this reason, members of the Native American Church are permitted to use peyote cactus, and, during liquor prohibition, churches and synagogues were allowed to continue to use wine. The religious-freedom clause of the First Amendment may, in the very near future, provide the only recourse by which longevists can protect their life-extension drugs and thus their own lives.

In 1971, a nondogmatic, nonprofit religious organization, known as the Church of the Tree of Life, was legally established in the United States. Its 6,000 members declared as their official sacraments numerous herbal and chemical substances that were still legal at the time. Included in its list of sacraments are most of the vitamins, nutritional components, and life-extension materials described in this book.

The Church requires only one belief of its members: that all adult human beings have the right to do with their own bodies, minds, and spirits whatever they wish, as long as their actions do not directly infringe on the rights of others. If the reader agrees with this philosophy and wishes to learn more about the Church, he can send $1 to cover the costs of materials and mailing to Church of the Tree of Life, 405 Columbus Avenue, San Francisco, CA 94133. If you mention that you learned of them through this book, they will include their special bulletin on life-extension techniques.

## The Last Word

I have not been able to discuss every factor that may relate to the extension of human lifespan or to mention every scientist who has made a worthy contribution to this pursuit; this is to be a book, not an encyclopaedia. But in looking over the completed manuscript, I realize that the names of several outstanding gerontologists are conspicuously absent. Among those are Elie Metchnikoff, Alexandr Bogomolets, Nathan Shock, and the late Fritz Verzár.

The Russian-born Metchnikoff won a Nobel Prize in 1908 for his pioneering work in immunology. He is most well-remembered, however, for his theories on intestinal detoxification. It was he who was mainly responsible for the popularity of yogurt in the Western world.

Bogomolets, another Russian and pupil of Metchnikoff, developed a biostimulant known as antireticular cytotoxic serum (ACS). This serum is produced by injecting connective tissues of young accident victims into animal bloodstreams and extracting the resultant antibodies. It is said to enhance immunologic responses, and thereby to assist healing, cure ailments, and extend lifespan. Although attempts to confirm or refute the efficacy of ACS in treating illness and injury have yielded varied and inconclusive results, it appears to have no measurable life-extending properties. Whatever the value of ACS may be, Bogomolets was probably the first scientist to bring attention to the relationship between the connective tissue and aging.

Dr. Shock, a noted physiologist and the director of NIH's Gerontological Research Center in Baltimore, Maryland, has deservedly been dubbed the dean of American gerontology. He has done significant work in measuring the effects of aging on various parts of the body and on the entire organism. He has collected and organized a staggering amount of gerontological literature from all corners of the scientific world, and has done much to lead the science of gerontology to where it stands today. He is also one of the leading proponents of several views that I have tried to emphasize throughout this book: that aging is a complex phenomenon requiring different explanatory principles for different aspects; that much of the process involves a breakdown of the endocrines and neural control mechanisms; and that research should give more attention to how aging affects the total organism, rather than to what happens to cells alone. Each month in the *Journal of Gerontology*, Dr. Shock publishes "Current Publications in Gerontology," in which he catalogs over 1,000 writings from books and journals about gerontology.

The Hungarian-born physician and physiologist Fritz Verzár made outstanding contributions in the fields of enzyme function, digestion, muscle function, and endocrinology. He also helped make experimental gerontology a respectable scientific discipline. After his mandatory retirement from the Institute of Physiology in Basel, Switzerland, at the age of 70, he continued his experiments on age changes in the connective tissues, established the Institute for Experimental Gerontology, and founded the journal *Gerontologia*. On March 12, 1979, at the age of 92, he passed away. His work and his enthusiasm were an inspiration to other gerontologists.

To these and other workers, living and dead, who seem to have been overlooked in this volume, and to those who have been mentioned only briefly, I would like to express my hope that I will be able to give them the full credit they deserve in future writings to be published in the *Quarterly Journal of the Megahealth Society*.

I suppose I might also be criticized for failing to emphasize the life-shortening hazards of such modern practices as smoking, excessive drinking, and drug abuse. However, since other books on health and life extension have devoted many pages to the effects of these noxious habits, and since their dangers are already well-known and well-documented, I see no need to dwell on these or any other avenues to suicide. Nevertheless, I would like to end this book by offering what I have found to be useful rules of thumb for life extension; and the reader may heed them or ignore them at his or her own risk.

Don't smoke.

Don't abuse drugs or alcohol.

Don't jump off tall buildings.

Don't overeat.

Don't consume refined carbohydrates.

Don't try to do too much at once.

Don't be a victim of retirement.

Don't become President of the United States. (Have you noticed how rapidly they age after taking office?)

Don't become overenthusiastic about the exciting things you have learned in this book. Don't postpone taking steps to improve your health; but also don't plunge recklessly into a full-blown life-extension program that uses every method and material described in this book.

Do be circumspect and approach new methods of life extension cautiously, with wisdom and with sensitivity to your body's responses.

Do learn to respond to your body's messages. Eat when you're hungry; stop when you're not; sleep when you're tired; etc.

Do set realistic goals.

Do steer clear of hectic schedules.

Do try to make your life worth living, and yourself worthy of life. If you feel that you have a right and reason to live long, you are more likely to do so.

Do what you can to make the world a better place to live in. If you are going to live 120 years or more, you don't want to do it on a nightmare planet.

Do try to keep abreast of the coming breakthroughs in gerontology.

Do take good care of yourself, and have a long and happy life.

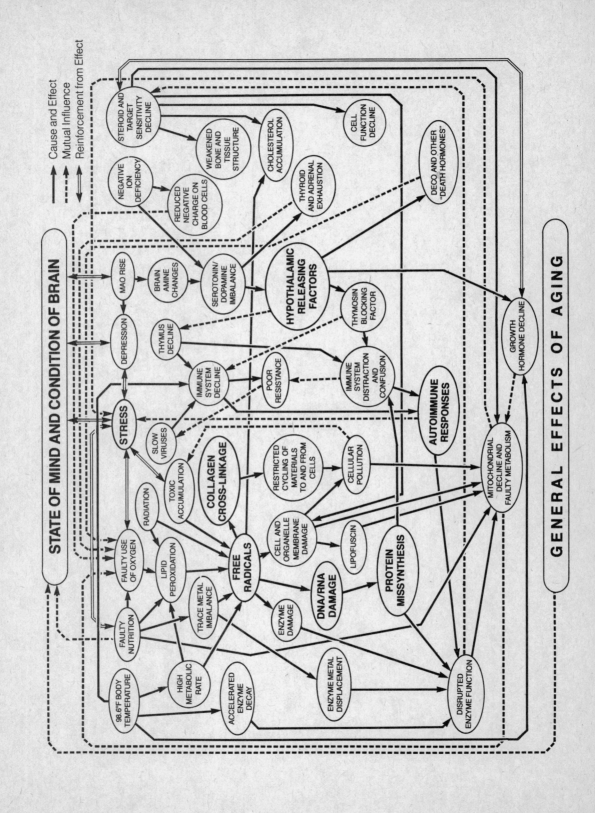

*How major causes of aging mutually increase each other's effects and accelerate the aging process.*

This chart synopsizes much of the information in this book, and shows how several contributing causes of aging do harm and potentiate each other's effects. The many intersecting lines and arrows may, at first glance, make the chart appear complex and difficult to comprehend. This appearance is partly intentional. It is meant to convey that aging appears to be caused or accelerated by several factors that depress normal biological functions, lead to further complications, and increase each other's harmful effects. As one studies the chart, however, its meanings should become more and more clear. One may begin with any single factor and, at a glance, see what other factors influence it, what factors it influences, and whether there is a direct or indirect mutually potentiating influence between it and any other factor. One may also follow sequences of events in which any one or several factors lead through a series of complications toward the ultimate degeneration of the body.

Starting at the top of the chart, one can see that state of mind and brain condition can have much influence over the general causes of aging and the rate at which the effects of aging progress. Following the dotted arrow from the bottom of the chart back to the top, one sees that the general effects of aging can, in turn, affect state of mind, and, consequently, the intensity of factors that contribute to aging. One can also see that certain factors, such as stress, depression, and faulty nutrition, can directly affect mental state. Reading from left to right, one can easily follow the chains of events that hasten senescence and death.

Hypothermia is the most effective experimental life-extension technique now known. Scientists predict that lowering the normal body temperature by only a few degrees could triple human lifespan. This would decrease both the general metabolic rate and the rate of enzyme decay. Hence, we may regard our normal 98.6°F temperature as inimical to the goal of long life. The more accelerated rate of enzyme decay disrupts enzyme functions. This results in faulty metabolism and a decline in the efficiency of the energy-producing mitochondria. These two complications not only are characteristic problems in aging, but also reinforce other causes of aging by contributing to stress and the faulty use of oxygen, as shown by the dotted arrows. The high metabolic rate from the 98.6°F internal temperature hastens the rates of lipid peroxidation and free-radical formation in the body, and these lead to several other complications which we will consider in a moment.

Faulty nutrition—especially insufficient dietary antioxidants, such as vitamins C and E—also increases lipid peroxidation and free radicals. It can also contribute to mitochondrial decline and faulty metabolism, and to faulty use of oxygen. This further amplifies the lipid-peroxidation/free-radical problem. If the diet fails to provide the required minerals, a trace-metal imbalance may occur, leading to enzyme-metal displacement (e.g., copper for zinc). This further disrupts enzyme functions, and this disruption further escalates the vicious cycle by increasing metabolic/mitochondrial failure, which leads back again to further stress, faulty oxygenation, lipid peroxidation, and free-radical proliferation.

Peroxidized lipids and free radicals cause harm in several ways: (1) they directly damage enzymes and disrupt their functions; (2) they damage DNA and RNA, which results in missynthesized protein and further disruption of enzyme functions; (3) they cause collagen cross-linkage, and cell and organelle membrane damage, which, among other things, leads to cellular pollution and reinforces the vicious cycle described above; (4) they increase the accumulation of cholesterol deposits on the arterial walls.

Both naturally occurring and man-proliferated radiation add to the free-radical problem. So do toxic accumulations, which are partly produced by stress.

Stress and faulty nutrition can be mutually potentiating factors, especially if dietary antistress agents are insufficient or if stress inhibits digestion and assimilation of nutrients. There are also mutual influences between stress and other factors.

The decreased output of the thymus leads to a functional decline in the immune system, resulting in increased autoimmune responses, poor resistance to disease, and greater susceptibility to certain slow-acting viruses that may be partly responsible for the aging phenomenon. If the immune system attacks the body's native protein, enzyme functions may become even more disrupted and further magnify the vicious cycle. Missynthesized proteins may increase the problem by confusing the immune system. Further decline of the immune system appears to be brought about by a thymosin-blocking factor that is secreted from the pituitary because of the influence of hypothalamic-releasing factors signaled by serotonin rises and dopamine declines. These changes also signal the release of DECO, which decreases the consumption of oxygen and again reinforces the vicious cycle that begins with faulty use of oxygen. It is believed that other "death hormones" are similarly released through the hypothalamic/pituitary axis. Negative-ion deficiency can also bring about the serotonin/dopamine disbalance, and add to the faulty-oxygenation problem by reducing the negative charge on the surface of red-blood-cell membranes. Overstimulation from too much serotonin can eventually exhaust the thyroid and adrenals, which still further reinforces the faulty use of oxygen.

A decline in the secretion of certain steroids, coupled with decreased target sensitivity to these hormones, produces many problems, including demineralization and weakening of bone and other tissue structure, increased cholesterol accumulation on the arterial walls, a general decline in cell functioning, and a loss of the protection that corticosteroids normally give to cell and organelle membranes.

Human Growth Hormone (HGH) may be one of the hypothesized "youth hormones." Hypothalamic-releasing factors influence its production in the pituitary during youth and its decrease in later life. Its decline diminishes the vitality of all tissues including those of the endocrines, and can inhibit both the production of steroids and the target sensitivity of the tissues to respond to them and to HGH. Reduced body temperatures slow down the decline of HGH, which brings us back to where we began with the 98.6°F internal body temperature.

# Antiaging Substances and Their Actions

| | ANTIOXIDANT/FREE-RADICAL DEACTIVATOR | ANTISTRESS AGENT | BRAIN-FUNCTION IMPROVER | DETOXIFYING AGENT | IMMUNE-SYSTEM IMPROVER | PROTEIN-SYNTHESIS IMPROVER | MEMBRANE STABILIZER | CARDIAC PROTECTOR | DNA REPAIR AID | ANTIBIOTIC AGENT | OXYGEN-USE FACTOR | Additional functions |
|---|---|---|---|---|---|---|---|---|---|---|---|---|
| Amygdalin | | | | | | | | • | | | | |
| Ascorbic Acid | • | • | | • | • | • | | • | • | | | |
| BAPN | | | | | | | | | | | | cross-linkage reverser |
| BHT – BHA | • | | | | | | | | | • | | |
| Biotin | | • | | | | • | | | • | | | |
| Calcium | | • | | | | | | | | | | |
| Centrophenoxine | • | | • | | | | • | | | | | lipofuscin decreaser |
| Choline | | | • | | | | | | • | | | |
| Chromium | | | | | | • | | • | • | | | |
| Cysteine | • | | | • | | • | | | • | | | |
| DMAE | • | | • | | | | | • | | | | lipofuscin decreaser |
| Folic Acid | | • | | | | • | | | • | | | |
| GH3 | | | • | • | | | | • | | | | hypothalamic-serotonin adjuster |
| Ginseng | | | • | | | | | | | | | |
| Inositol | | | | | | | | • | | | | |
| L-dopa | | | | | | | | | | | | hypothalamic-serotonin adjuster |
| Lecithin | • | | • | | | | | | | | | |
| Magnesium | | • | | | | | | • | | | | |
| Manganese | | | • | | | | | • | • | | • | |
| 2-MEA | • | | | • | • | • | | | | | | |
| Methionine | • | | | • | | • | | | • | | | lipotropic agent |
| Molybdenum | | | | | | | | | • | | | |

# Antiaging Substances and Their Actions, *cont.*

| | ANTIOXIDANT/FREE-RADICAL DEACTIVATOR | ANTISTRESS AGENT | BRAIN-FUNCTION IMPROVER | DETOXIFYING AGENT | IMMUNE-SYSTEM IMPROVER | PROTEIN-SYNTHESIS IMPROVER | MEMBRANE STABILIZER | CARDIAC PROTECTOR | DNA REPAIR AID | ANTIBIOTIC AGENT | OXYGEN-USE FACTOR | |
|---|---|---|---|---|---|---|---|---|---|---|---|---|
| Niacin | | • | • | | | • | | • | | | • | |
| Nucleic Acids | | | | | | • | | | • | | | |
| Orotic Acid | | | | | | | | | • | | | |
| PABA | • | • | | | | | • | | | | | UV screen |
| Pangamic Acid | | • | | • | | | | • | | | • | |
| Pantothenic Acid | | • | • | | | • | | | • | | | |
| Penicillamine | | | | • | | | | | | • | | cross-linkage reverser |
| PUFA | | | | | | | | • | | | | |
| Pyridoxine | | • | | | | • | | | • | | | |
| Riboflavin | | • | | | | | | | • | | | |
| Selenium | • | | | • | • | | | • | | | | |
| Sulfadiazine | | | | | | | | | | • | | |
| Thiamine | • | • | | | | | | | • | | • | |
| Thiodipropionate | • | | | | | | | | | | | |
| Thymosin | | | | | • | | | | | | | |
| Vitamin A | • | | | | | | • | • | | | • | |
| Vitamin E | • | | | | • | | • | • | • | | • | |
| Zinc | | | • | | • | • | | • | • | | | |

# Chapter Thirteen
# Life-Extension Directory

## *Appendix A*
### Supply Sources

Most of the materials needed for a life-extension program are both universally legal and easily available. But some are not legally or easily obtainable in some areas, or are otherwise difficult to locate. For these, some indications of supply sources are here provided.

### Selenium

Brewer's yeast can be a rich source of selenium (50 to 100 mcg per tablespoonful) if the mineral is present in the culture medium on which the yeast is grown. Many brands of yeast contain selenium, but do not mention it on the label. Among the few that do are Three Star Brand Selenium 600 Nutritional Yeast and Dr. Donsbach's (RichLife, Inc.) Yeast 500. At present, these cost around three or four dollars a pound. Like most yeasts, they are also rich sources of B vitamins, protein, and nucleic acids. Most health stores now carry 50-mcg tablets of selenium derived from yeast. Prices range between two and six dollars per 100 tablets.

Selenium ascorbate, a molecular combination of selenium and vitamin C, is an easily assimilated form of the mineral. It is produced by Alacer Corporation, at 100 50-mcg tablets for $3.95. They are available at many health-food stores, or may be ordered directly from the manufacturer, which also produces many other mineral ascorbates. Their address is 7425-C Orangethorpe Avenue, Buena Park, CA 90621. For their catalog, send 25¢ to cover handling costs.

Some longevists obtain sodium selenite from chemical suppliers and prepare a liquid concentrate from it, which they add as drops to drinking water and beverages. This is an excellent source of the mineral, but unless you know exactly how to prepare and use it, overdosage may occur. For this reason, we cannot recommend sodium selenate for the average reader. For complete information about its preparation and use, see *Quarterly Journal of the Megahealth Society*, 1 (1980), 7.

### Vitamins

Ascorbic acid, vitamin E acetate, cysteine hydrochloride, ethoxyquin, BHT, thiodipropionic acid, dilauryl thiodipropionate, and many other vitamins, antioxidants, and related materials are available at extraordinarily low prices from Vitamin Research Products, 1954-C2 Old Middlefield Way, Mountain View, CA 94043. To obtain their price list, send them a SASE or 25¢ to cover mailing. Their products are sold in bulk, powdered form, in quantities of 25, 50, 100, 250, 500, and 1,000 grams. When ordering, do not ask for information on recommended dosages or effects of these vitamins and drugs. FDA rulings do not permit producers and suppliers to offer such information, since this would constitute claims about the effects of the products. Such questions should be directed to the Megahealth Information Center (see page 160).

Pangamic acid (vitamin B15) is sold in some health stores, or can be ordered from any of the following companies:

Food Science Laboratories, Inc., South Burlington, VT 05401.

Natural Nutritional, P.O. Box 448, Passaic, NJ 07055.
Nutridyn Products Corp., 5705 West Howard St.,
Niles, IL 60648.

## Ion Generators

Several companies are now selling reasonably priced
negative-ion generators through some health-food
stores and by mail order. Because of FDA rulings, they
are not permitted to make any specific health claims for
the devices in their advertising and informational literature. The interested reader should request brochures
from each of the companies listed below, and compare
the products and prices. Enclose $1 to cover handling
costs.

Cosmic Creations, 1255 Montgomery Street, San
    Francisco, CA 94133; (415) 956-0654.
B & B Specialties, 16702 Cherry Ave., Torrance, CA
    90504; (213) 323-2288.
Cheops, 8143-F Big Bend, Webster Groves, MO
    63119.
JS&A National Sales Group, One JS&A Plaza, North-
    brook, IL 60062. Call toll-free (800) 323-6400. In
    Illinois, call (312) 564-7000.

One can obtain 2-mercaptoethylamine and 4-thi-
azolidinecarboxylic acid may be obtained from
several chemical companies, including Calbiochem-
Behring, Box 12087, San Diego, CA 92112. Since the
available forms of these two chemicals are not graded
as pure enough for human consumption, we cannot
legally recommend their use. Some self-experimenters
hold that the impurities in these chemicals (laboratory
grade, rather than pharmaceutical grade) are so minute
that, although they do not pass FDA requirements,
they contain fewer impurities than our most untainted
foods. Since fairly low-milligram dosages of the drugs
are used, laboratory grades are probably safe for oral
use, but they are too impure for injection.

## GH3 and Procaine

Until recently, GH3 therapy has not been available to
the general public in the United States. The only way
that Americans could receive treatments was to go to
Romania. Now, the government ruling has been
changed to allow GH3 therapy in the state of Nevada.
Since August 1, 1978, Rom-American Pharmaceuticals, Ltd., now in Las Vegas, has been permitted to
produce oral GH3 in capsules. They plan soon to
manufacture an injectable form of the drug. Both of
these will be available by prescription only, through
physicians and pharmacies in Nevada. They will not
be available in other states, unless the ruling is further
changed, and cannot be shipped across state lines. For
information, write to Rom-American Pharmaceuticals, Ltd., 300 South 4th Street, Las Vegas, NV
89109, or telephone (702) 386-0397.

GH3 therapy is also available in Mexico at Lake
Chapala, just south of Guadalajara. For information
and reservations, write to Touch of Eden, 2401 East
Washington Blvd., Pasadena, CA 91104, or phone
(213) 798-0701. Those who wish to go to one of Dr.
Aslan's own clinics in Romania can arrange package
tours through any Romanian tourist office, or by con-
tacting the Carpati National Tourist Office, Magheru
Blvd., Bucharest 7, Romania.

Procaine hydrochloride is available legally from
many chemical companies. Because of this, some
longevists may want to attempt self-administration. We
do not recommend this, however. Although procaine
is very nontoxic, some individuals can have allergic
reactions to it. The drug should only be taken under
the supervision of a physician.

We have been informed that Gerovital is now sold
in Mexican pharmacies without prescription, and that
some people obtain it in Tijuana and bring it back to
the United States. This is not advisable, since customs
officials would not take kindly to anyone caught smug-
gling even small amounts for personal use.

## Cell Therapy

For information on treatment at the clinic founded by
Niehans, write to Dr. Walter Michel, Director, Cli-
nique La Prairie, Clarens-Montreaux, 1820 Switzerland, or telephone Switzerland, 021-62-43-77.

For information on fresh-cell therapy at a West
German clinic, write to Dr. Siegfried Blöck, Director,
Privatsanatorium für Frischzellen-Behandlung,
D-8172 Lenggries/Obb, Latschenkopfstrasse 2, Federal
Republic of Germany, or telephone West Germany
0-80-42-83-25.

There are two sources of information on fresh-
frozen-cell therapy in the American continent: Dr.
George Vlassis, Director, Avenida Paseo Tijuana 103,
Playas de Tijuana, Mexico, or, for appointments
through their San Diego office, telephone (714)
426-3603, ext. 8; and Dr. Ivan M. Popov, Medical
Director, Renaissance Clinic, Balmoral Beach, Box
128, Nassau, Bahamas, or telephone Nassau 77481.

## Herbs

Ginseng, *gotu kola*, and fleeceflower tubers may be
sold by your local herb dealer, or they can be mail-
ordered from Magic Garden Herb Co., P.O. Box 332,
Fairfax, CA 94140. Live *gotu kola* plants can be
ordered from Thomas A. David, Independent Scientific Research, 19886 Geer Ave., Hilmar, CA 95324.
Enclose 25¢ when requesting catalogs from either of
these companies.

# *Appendix B*
## Life-Extension Publications and Organizations

It has not been possible to cover here every known facet of life extension. Furthermore, new discoveries are constantly being reported. Even while I was writing this book, I had to make numerous revisions to accommodate recent findings. The reader who wishes to keep abreast of new information can subscribe to the *Quarterly Journal of the Megahealth Society*, which includes information on life extension, nutrition, attaining superior states of health, increasing intelligence, healing techniques, and many other related subjects. Single issues are $2. One year's subscription is $7. Our address is: Megahealth Society, P.O. Box 1684, Manhattan Beach, CA 90266. We also welcome questions for the "Question and Answer Forum" in our journal. These should be typed and as brief as possible. If a personal response is desired, the question must include a self-addressed envelope with postage.

Some of the other life-extension groups listed here also publish periodicals or bulletins to which the reader may wish to subscribe. Any similar groups whom we have omitted are invited to contact the Megahealth Society, so that we can mention them in our quarterly journal and in future editions of this book. When requesting information from the organizations listed here, include $1 to cover costs of materials and mailing.

Aging Prevention Research Foundation, Ltd., 216 Sea Cliff Ave., Sea Cliff, NY 11579. Telephone: (516) 671-8790. Ray Prohaska, Founder-Director.

Alcor Life-Extension Foundation, P.O. Box 312, Glendale, CA 91209. Telephone: (213) 956-6042. Laurence Gale, President.

American Aging Association, University of Nebraska Medical Center, 42d and Dewey Ave., Omaha, NE 68015. Telephone: (402) 541-4000. Denham Harman, Director. this group publishes *AGE News*, a quarterly journal, and holds an annual symposium, which is later published by Raven Press.

Biofutures, 840 S.E. 22nd Ave., Apt. 4-B, Pompano Beach, FL 33062. Telephone: (305) 735-5556.

The Committee for the Elimination of Death, P.O. Box 696, San Marcos, CA 92069. A. Stuart Otto, Chairman.

The Foundation for Aging Research, 6961 Valjean Ave., Van Nuys, CA 91406. Telephone: (213) 782-4251. Dr. Benjamin Schloss, Director.

Foundation for Infinite Survival, Inc., P.O. Box 4000-C, Berkeley, CA 94704. Chadd A. Everone,

Governing Trustee. Among other things, they offer multiphasic medical examinations at their Health Testing Center.

International Association on the Artificial Prolongation of Human Specific Lifespan, Fabiolalaan, 12 Knokke-Zoute, B-8300, Belgium, publishes *Rejuvenation*, a journal containing articles in English and French.

Live Longer Now Center, P.O. Box 26723, 109 South Scott Ave., Tucson, AZ 85726. Telephone: (602) 888-4188. Jon N. Leonard, Director.

Long Life Magazine (formerly *Life Extension*), 663 W. Barry, Chicago, IL 60657. Bimonthly journal. Single issue, $3; 1-year subscription, $12; 2 years, $22; 3 years, $33. Canada, add $2 a year; foreign countries (not U.S. possessions), add $6 a year.

Man's Frontiers Foundation, Inc., P.O. Box 636, Sandy Hook, CT 06482. Herbert Bailey, Director.

The Network, P.O. Box 317, Berkeley, CA 94701.

Pauling Institute of Science and Medicine, 2700 Sandy Hill, Menlo Park, CA 94025. Telephone: (415) 854-0843. Linus Pauling, Director. Dues of $15 a year contribute to Dr. Pauling's important research on ascorbic acid, make you a member of the Friends of Linus Pauling Institute, and entitle you to receive their quarterly bulletin and other literature.

Prometheus Society, Inc., 102 Morris Drive, Laurel, MD 20810. Charles E. Tandy, Founding Director.

Those who are interested in cryonic suspension can contact any of the following organizations:

The Alcor Society for Solid State Hypothermia, Box 312, Glendale, CA 91209. Telephone: (213) 956-6042. Allen McDaniels, President.

Bay Area Cryonics Society, 7710 Huntridge Lane, Cupertino, CA 95014. Telephone: (415) 763-6647. Jerome White, President.

The Cryonics Association, 24041 Stratford, Oak Park, MI 48237. Telephone: (313) 398-6624. Robert C. W. Ettinger, President.

The Cryonics Society of Australia, Box 18, O'Connor ACT 2600, Australia.

Cryonics Society of San Diego, 4791 50th St., San Diego, CA 92115. Cdr. Loren Fitzgerald, President.

Cryonics Society of Southern Florida, Inc., 2835 Hollywood Blvd., Hollywood, FL 33020. Telephone: (305) 925-2500. Steven Rievman, President.

Hartman Help, Inc., Stuart, IA 50250. Telephone: (515) 279-6649 (C-R-Y-O-N-I-X)

Trans Time, Inc., 1122 Spruce St., Berkeley, CA 94707. Telephone: (415) 525-7114. Arthur Quaife, President.

# Recommended Reading

Bailey, Herbert. *GH3: Will It Keep You Young Longer?* N.Y.: Bantam, 1977. Good study of aging theories with emphasis on Gerovital therapy. Appendix contains 25 papers from scientific literature.

Comfort, Alex. *Ageing: The Biology of Senescence.* London: Routledge & Kegan Paul, 1964. Early, but interesting and intelligent study by gerontologist turned popular writer and sexologist.

Frank, Benjamin S., with Philip Miele. *Dr. Frank's No-Aging Diet.* N.Y.: Dell, 1976. Easily read study of deterioration in aging, and of its control by means of nucleic acid therapy.

Kent, Saul. *The Life-Extension Revolution.* N.Y.: William Morrow, 1979. Up-to-date reviews of major findings in gerontology with suggested approaches to better health and longer life. One of the most highly recommended studies.

Kugler, Hans J. *Slowing Down the Aging Process.* N.Y.: Pyramid, 1973. Good information on controlling aging, primarily by means of improved nutrition.

Kurtzman, Joel, and Gordon, P. *No More Dying.* N.Y.: Dell, 1976. Popular review of gerontology.

Lindsay, Rae. *The Pursuit of Youth.* N.Y.: Pinnacle Books, 1976. Popular study of antiaging therapies and cosmetic surgery. Gives addresses of many spas and clinics throughout the world.

McGrady, Patrick. *The Youth Doctors.* N.Y.: Coward-McCann, 1968. Older, but informative work about theories and therapies. Contains many photographs.

Passwater, Richard A. *Supernutrition.* N.Y.: Pocket Books, 1976. The use of megavitamins for better health and longer life. Dosage tables and charts included.

Prehoda, Robert W. *Extended Youth.* N.Y.: Putnam's, 1968. Pioneering work on aging theories and life extension. Although now outdated in places, it contains much useful information and thoughtful speculation.

Rockstein, Morris, *et al.*, eds. *Theoretical Aspects of Aging.* N.Y.: Academic Press, 1974. Symposium-derived anthology; fourteen chapters by leading gerontologists.

Rosenfeld, Albert. *Prolongevity.* N.Y.: Knopf, 1976. Thoughtful and fairly up-to-date work by highly esteemed science writer.

Segerberg, Osborn, Jr. *The Immortality Factor.* N.Y.: Dutton/Bantam, 1974/1975. Detailed study of man's search for immortality through the ages and up to recent times.

Selye, Hans. *The Stress of Life.* N.Y.: McGraw-Hill, 1956. Early but worthwhile treatise about effects of stress on health and lifespan; by major researcher.

Strehler, Bernard L. *Time, Cells, and Aging.* N.Y.: Academic Press, 2d ed., 1977. Most useful and authoritative work about entropic processes of aging on cellular, molecular, and genetic levels; by a foremost gerontologist.

Winter, Ruth. *Ageless Aging.* N.Y.: Crown, 1973. Informative and easily read work by popular science writer.

# References

1. Abrams, A., *et al.*, *J. Gerontol.*, 20 (1965), 139.
2. Ahrens, E., *et al.*, *J. Exp. Med.*, 90 (1949), 409.
3. Asdell, S. A., *et al.*, *J. Reprod. Fert.*, 14 (1967), 113.
4. Aslan, A., *Die Therapiewoche*, 7 (1956), 14.
5. Aslan, A., *et al.*, *Fiziol. Norm. Pat.*, 18 (1972), 81.
6. Aslan, A., in *Theoretical Aspects of Aging*, M. Rockstein *et al.*, eds. (New York: Academic Press, 1974), p. 145.
7. Bailey, H., *Vitamin E: Your Key to a Healthy Heart* (New York: Arco, 1971).
8. Bailey, H., *GH3: Will It Keep You Young Longer?* (New York: Bantam, 1977), p. 108.
9. Bang, F. B., *et al.*, *Fed. Proc.*, 36 (1977), 3.
10. Barrows, C. H., *Gerontologist*, 11 (1971), 5.
11. Bell, E., *et al.*, *Science*, 202 (1978), 1158.
12. Bellamy, D., *Symp. Soc. Expl Biol.*, 21 (1967), 427.
13. Bellamy, D., *Expl Gerontol.*, 3 (1968), 327.
14. Bender, A. D., *et al.*, *Expl Gerontol.*, 5 (1970), 97.
15. Benedict, J. D., *et al.*, *Metabolism*, 1 (1952), 3.
16. Berryman, J. A. W., *et al.*, *Brit. Med. J.*, 526S (1961), 1683.
17. Bernstein, T. F., *Zdravookhr. Beloruss.*, 18, No. 10 (1972), 34.
18. Birch, T. W., *et al.*, *Nature*, 138 (1936), 27.
19. Birnberg, C. H., and R. Kurzrok, *J. Amer. Geriat. Soc.*, 3 (1955), 656.
20. Bjorksten, J., *Chem. Industries*, 48 (1941), 746.
21. Bjorksten, J., *Chem. Industries*, 50 (1942), 68.
22. Bjorksten, J., *J. Amer. Geriat. Soc.*, 16 (1968), 408.
23. Bjorksten, J., *Miami Symposium on Theoretical Aspects of Aging* (Feb. 7, 1974).
24. Black, H. S., and J. T. Chan, *Food Cosmet. Toxicol.*, 11 (1973), 199.
25. Ulland, B. M., *et al.*, *J. Invest. Dermatol.*, 65 (1975), 412.
26. Bodansky, M., and S. L. Engel, *Nature*, 210 (1966), 751.
27. Bodenstein, D., *J. Expl Zool.*, 129 (1955), 209.
28. Bowman, R. E., *Science*, 153 (1966), 902.
29. Boynton, H., *Bestways* (Sept. 1976), p. 36.
30. Brekhman, I. I., and I. V. Dardymov, *Ann. Rev. Pharmacol.*, 9 (1969), 419.
31. Brooks, D. M., III, *Libertarian Connection*, no. 73 (1977), p. 5.
32. Brown, P. E., *Nature*, 213 (1967), 363.
33. Brugh, M., Jr., *Science*, 197 (Sept. 23, 1977), 1291.
34. Bunag, R. D., and E. J. Walaszek, *Arch. Intern. Pharmacodyn.*, 135 (1962), 142.
35. Buu-Hoi, N. P., and A. R. Ratsimamanga, *Comptes Rendus des Séances Soc. Biol.*, 153 (1959), 1180.
36. Caldwell, B. M., *J. Gerontol.*, 9 (1954), 168.
37. Callahan, E. J. *et al.*, *Med. Rec.*, 149 (1939), 167.
38. Carpenter, D. G., and J. A. Loynd, *J. Amer. Geriat. Soc.*, 16 (1968), 1307.
39. Meier-Ruge, W., *et al.*, *Fed. Proc.*, 32 (1973), 728; Abstract 2904.
40. Charman, R. C., *et al.*, *Angiol.*, 23 (1973), 29.
41. Cherkin, A., at *State-of-the-Art Workshop on "Procaine and Related Geropharmacologic Agents,"* V.A. Central Office, Washington, D.C. (Feb. 14, 1975).
42. Chio, K. S., and A. L. Tappel, *Biochem.*, 8 (1969), 2827.
43. Comfort, A., *The Process of Aging* (New York: Signet/NAL, 1964), p. 16.
44. Comfort, A., *et al.*, *Nature*, 229 (1971), 254.
45. Committee on Animal Nutrition, *Nutrient Requirements for Laboratory Animals* (Pub. No. 990, National Academy of Science).
46. Cone, C. D., Jr., *Proc. 12th Ann. Sci. Writers' Sem. of Amer. Cancer Soc.*, San Antonio, Texas (March, 1970).
47. Cotzias, G., *Proc. Nat. Acad. Sci.*, 71 (1974), 2466.
48. Cotzias, G., *Science*, 196 (1977), 549.
49. Cowan, D. W., *et al.*, *J. Amer. Med. Assn*, 120 (1942), 1268.
50. Crawford, M. A., *Lancet*, 1 (1962), 352.
51. Pfeiffer, C. C., *Zinc and Other Micronutrients* (New Canaan, CT: Keats, 1978), Chap. 18.

52. Cristalfo, V. J., *Adv. Gerontol. Res.*, 4 (1972), 105.
53. Curtis, H. J., *Gerontologist*, 6 (1966), 143.
54. Cutting, W. C., *Handbook of Pharmacology* (New York: Appleton-Century-Crofts, 5th ed., 1972), pp. 114–115.
55. *Ibid.*, p. 158.
56. *Ibid.*, pp. 161–162.
57. *Ibid.*, pp. 251–252.
58. *Ibid.*, p. 408.
59. *Ibid.*, p. 597.
60. Danes, B. S., *J. Clin. Invest.*, 50 (1971), 2000.
61. d'Aureous, S., *Libertarian Connection*, no. 72 (1977), p. 8.
62. Davis, A., *Let's Eat Right to Keep Fit* (New York: Signet, 1970), Chap. 7.
63. *Ibid.*, Chap. 9.
64. *Ibid.*, Chap. 10.
65. *Ibid.*, Chap. 11.
66. *Ibid.*, Chap. 12.
67. *Ibid.*, Chap. 17.
68. *Ibid.*, Chap. 18.
69. *Ibid.*, Chap. 19.
70. *Ibid.*, Chap. 20.
71. *Ibid.*, Chap. 21.
72. *Ibid.*, Chap. 22.
73. *Ibid.*, Chap. 23.
74. Davis, A., *Let's Get Well* (New York: Signet, 1972), Chap. 10.
75. *Ibid.*, Chap. 12.
76. *Ibid.*, Chap. 18.
77. *Ibid.*, Chap. 20.
78. *Ibid.*, Chap. 32.
79. Dawn, L., *Vitamins and Food Additives*. Available for $1.00 from L. Dawn, Box 90913, Worldway Postal Center, Los Angeles, CA 90009.
80. Denckla, W. D., *J. Clin. Invest.*, 53 (1974), 572.
81. Denckla, W. D., and G. E. Bilder, *Mech. Aging Devel.*, 6 (1977), 153.
82. DiCyan, E., *Vitamin E and Aging* (New York: Pyramid, 1972).
83. DiPalma, J. R., and D. M. Ritchie, *Ann. Rev. Pharmacol. Toxicol.*, 7 (1977), 133.
84. Donaldson, T., *Libertarian Connection*, no. 72 (1977), p. 6.
85. Donaldson, T., *Life Extension* (Mar./Apr. 1977), p. 3.
86. Donaldson, T., *Long Life* (Nov./Dec. 1977), p. 132.
87. Drenick, E. J., *et al.*, *J. Amer. Med. Assn*, 187 (1964), 100.
88. Duvoisin, R. C., *Trans. Amer. Neurol. Assn*, 94 (1969), 81.
89. Eddy, D., and D. Harman, *Fourth Ann. Meet. Amer. Aging Assn*, Los Angeles (Sept. 21, 1974).
90. Elam, L. H., and H. T. Blumenthal, in *Interdisciplinary Topics of Gerontology* (New York: Karger, 1970).
91. Ellis, D. B., *et al.*, *Life Sci.*, 7 (1968), 1259.
92. Emmenegger, H., and W. Meier-Ruge, *Pharmacol.*, 1 (1968), 65.
93. Enz, A., *et al.*, *Triangle*, 14, no. 2 (1975), 90.
94. Everitt, A. V., *Gerontologia*, 3 (1959), 37.

95. Everitt, A. V., *J. Gerontol.*, 14 (1959), 415.
96. Everitt, A. V., *J. Gerontol.*, 23 (1968), 333.
97. *Fed. Reg.* (July 9, 1965).
98. Fee, S. R., and A. N. G. Clark, *Brit. Med. J.*, 526S (1961), 1680.
99. Feldman, E. B., in *Niacin in Vascular Disorders and Hyperlipemia*, R. Altschul, ed. (Springfield, Ill.: Chas. C. Thomas, 1964), p. 208.
100. Földi, M. *et al.*, *Deutsche Gesellschaft für Gerontologie*, 3 (1970), 97.
101. Foulds, W. S., *et al.*, *Lancet*, 1 (1970), 35.
102. Foy, J. M., and J. R. Parratt, *Lancet*, 1 (1962), 942.
103. Frank, B. S., *A New Approach to Degenerative Disease and Aging* (New York: Patria Press, 1964).
104. Frank, B. S., *Nucleic-Acid Therapy in Aging and Degenerative Disease* (Lisbon, Port.: Fiquima, 3d ed., 1975).
105. Frank, B. S., and P. Miele, *Dr. Frank's No-Aging Diet* (New York: Dell, 1976).
106. Freedman, D. X., and N. J. Giarman, *Ann. N.Y. Acad. Sci.*, 96 (1962), 98.
107. Freedman, D. X., *Amer. J. Psychiat.*, 119 (1963), 843.
108. Freeman, C. K., *Biophys. Res. Comn.*, 4 (1973), 1573.
109. Friedman, H. *et al.*, *Nature*, 205 (1965), 1050.
110. Friedman, S. M., and C. L. Friedman, *Nature*, 200 (1963), 237.
111. Friedman, S. M., and C. L. Friedman, *Expl Gerontol.*, 1 (1964), 37.
112. Fulder, S. J., *Expl Gerontol.*, 12 (1977), 125.
113. Gardner, T. S., *J. Gerontol.*, 1 (1946), 445.
114. Gerras, C., ed., *The Complete Book of Vitamins* (Emmaus, Pa.: Rodale Press, 1977), p. 218.
115. *Ibid.*, pp. 648–649.
116. *Ibid.*, Chaps. 33 and 34.
117. Gitman, L., *et al.*, *Fifth Internatl Congr. Gerontol.*, San Francisco, Abstr. (1961), 54.
118. Glasky, A. T., and L. N. Simon, *Science*, 151 (1966), 702.
119. Goldstein, A., in *Advances in Metabolic Disorders*, Vol. 5 (New York: Academic Press, 1971).
120. Goldstein, A., and A. White, in *Contemporary Topics in Immunology* (New York: Plenum Press, 1973).
121. Goldstein, B. D., *et al.*, *Arch. Environ. Health*, 24 (1972), 243.
122. Gottlieb, A., *Sex Drugs and Aphrodisiacs* (Berkeley, Calif.: And/Or Press, 1974), pp. 35–38.
123. Groth, D. F., *et al.*, *J. Pharm. Expl Therap.*, 122 (1950), 20A.
124. Guillemin, R., and R. Burgus, *Sci. Amer.* (Nov. 1972), p. 24.
125. Hackmann, C., *Experientia*, 18 (1962), 476.
126. Hadjimarkos, D. M., *Food Cosmet. Toxicol.*, 11 (1973), 1083.
127. Hall, N., *Libertarian Connection*, no. 67 (1977), p. 5.
128. Hall, N., *Libertarian Connection*, no. 70 (1977), p. 1.
129. Hall, N., and S. d'Aureous, *Libertarian Connection*, no. 73 (1977), p. 2.
130. Harman, D., *J. Gerontol.*, 11 (1956), 298.
131. Harman, D., *J. Gerontol.*, 12 (1957), 257.

132. Harman, D., *J. Gerontol.*, 16 (1961), 247.
133. Harman, D., *Radiat. Res.*, 16 (1962), 753.
134. Harman, D., *Gerontologist*, 8 (1968), 13.
135. Harman, D., *J. Gerontol.*, 23 (1968), 476.
136. Harman, D., *Ann. Meet. Gerontol. Soc.*, (1972).
137. Harman, D., *J. Amer. Geriat. Soc.* (April 20, 1972), 145.
138. Hawkins, D., and L. Pauling, eds., *Orthomolecular Psychiatry: Treatment of Schizophrenia* (San Francisco: W. H. Freeman, 1973).
139. Hayflick, L., and P. S. Moorhead, *Expl Cell Res.*, 25 (1961), 585.
140. Hayflick, L., *Sci. Amer.* (Mar. 1968), p. 218.
141. Henneman, D. H., *Endocrin.*, 83 (1968), 678.
142. Himwich, W. A., and E. Costa, *Fed. Proc.*, 19 (1960), 838.
143. Hirsh, J., *Brit. Med. J.*, 526S (1961), 1684.
144. Hochschild, R., *Expl Gerontol.*, 8 (1973), 185.
145. Hochschild, R., *Gerontologia*, 19 (1973), 271.
146. Hochschild, R., at *State-of-the-Art Workshop on "Procaine and Related Geropharmacologic Agents,"* V.A. Central Office, Washington, D.C. (Feb. 14, 1975).
147. Hodges, R. E., and E. M. Baker, in *Modern Nutrition in Health and Disease*, R. S. Goodhart and M. E. Shils, eds. (Philadelphia: Lea & Febiger, 5th ed., 1973), p. 253.
148. Hoffer, A., *Niacin Therapy in Psychiatry* (Springfield, Ill.: Chas. C. Thomas, 1962).
149. Hoffer, A., and H. Osmond, *How to Live with Schizophrenia* (New Hyde Park, N.Y.: University Books, 1966).
150. Hoffer, A., and H. Osmond, *The Hallucinogens* (New York and London: Academic Press, 1967), p. 28.
151. *Ibid.*, pp. 212, 215, and 216.
152. *Ibid.*, p. 217.
153. *Ibid.*, p. 309.
154. *Ibid.*, p. 312.
155. *Ibid.*, pp. 503–508.
156. *Ibid.*, p. 507.
157. *Ibid.*, Chaps. II-A and IV.
158. Holland, J. J., *Sci. Amer.* (Feb. 1974), p. 32.
159. Holliday, R., *et al.*, *Science*, 198 (Oct. 28, 1977), 366.
160. Hopkins, L. L., Jr., and H. E. Mohr, *Fed. Proc.*, 33 (1974), 1773.
161. Hoppe, J. O., *et al.*, *Amer. J. Med. Sci.*, 230 (1955), 558.
162. Hornykiewics, O., *Pharmacol. Rev.*, 18 (1966), 925.
163. Hruza, Z., *Expl Gerontol.*, 2 (1967), 201.
164. Hruza, Z., *Expl Gerontol.*, 6 (1971), 103.
165. Hsu, T. H., *et al.*, *Proc. Soc. Expl Biol. Med.*, 143 (1973), 577.
166. Hunter, H., *Bestways* (May 1978), p. 23.
167. Iwangoff, P., *et al.*, *Pharmacol.*, 14 (1976), 27.
168. Jacobson, E., *Anxiety and Tension Control* (Philadelphia, Pa.: Lippincott, 1964).
169. *J. Amer. Med. Assn*, 184 (1963), 992.
170. *Ibid.*, 215, Questions and Answers (1971), 292.
171. Kalz, F., *Arch. Dermat.*, 78 (1958), 740.
172. Kao, K.-Y., *et al.*, *Proc. Soc. Expl Biol. Med.*, 119 (1965), 364.
173. Karlow, W., *J. Pharmacol. and Expl Therap.*, 104 (1952), 122.
174. Kemeny, G., and B. Rosenberg, *Nature*, 253 (1973), 400.
175. Kent, J. R., and A. B. Agone, in *Androgens in Normal and Pathological Conditions*. A. Vermeulen, ed. (Amsterdam, Neth.: Exerpta Medica Foundation, 1966), p. 31.
176. Kent, S., *Life Extension* (July/Aug. 1977), p. 77.
177. Kirschmann, J. D., *Nutrition Almanac* (New York: McGraw-Hill, 1975), p. 91.
178. *Ibid.*, p. 92.
179. Kittler, G. D., *Laetrile: Control for Cancer* (New York: Warner, 1963).
180. Klerman, G. L., *J. Psychiat. Res.*, 9 (1972), 253.
181. Kment, A., in *Zellforschung und Zelltherapie*, F. Schmid and J. Stein, eds. (Bern, Switz.: Hans Huber, 1963).
182. Kohn, R. R., and A. M. Leash, *Expl Mol. Path.*, 1 (1967), 354.
183. Konigsmark, B. W., and E. A. Murphy, *Nature*, 288 (1970), 1335.
184. Kopin, I. J., in *Drugs and the Brain*. P. Black, ed. (Baltimore, Md.: Johns Hopkins, 1969), p. 3.
185. Krebs, E. T., Jr., ed and transl., *Vitamin B₁₅ (Pangamic Acid): Properties, Functions, and Uses*, from U.S.S.R. anthol. (Montreal, Que., Can.: McNaughton Foundation, 1966).
186. Kreuger, A. P., *Internat. J. Biometeor.*, 12 (1968), 225.
187. Kreuger, R. G., *et al.*, *Introduction to Microbiology* (New York: Macmillan, 1973), Part 6.
188. Kugler, H. J., *Slowing Down the Aging Process* (New York: Pyramid, 1973), pp. 71, 148, and 173.
189. *Ibid.*, p. 130.
190. *Ibid.*, p. 137.
191. *Ibid.*, p. 138.
192. *Ibid.*, pp. 140–141.
193. *Ibid.*, p. 146.
194. *Ibid.*, p. 152.
195. *Ibid.*, Chaps. 2 and 3.
196. *Ibid.*, Chap. 11.
197. Kugler, H. J., *American Laboratory*, 8 (Nov. 1976), 24.
198. Kurtzman, J., and P. Gordon, *No More Dying* (New York: Dell, 1976), p. 135.
199. *Ibid.*, p. 138.
200. *Ibid.*, p. 183.
201. Kysor, G., *Libertarian Connection*, no. 72 (1977), p. 3.
202. Labecki, T. D., *Amer. J. Clin. Nutr.*, 6 (1958), 325.
203. LaBella, F., *Gerontologist*, 8 (1968), 13.
204. LaBella, F. S., in *Search for New Drugs*, A. A. Rubin, ed. (New York: Marcel Dekker, 1972), p. 347.
205. Leith, J. D., Jr., *Gerontologist*, 7 (1967), 244.
206. Levander, O. A., *J. Amer. Diet. Assn*, 66 (1975), 338.
207. Levander, O. A., *Fed. Proc.*, 36 (1977), 1683.
208. Li, C.-H., and D. Yamashiro, *J. Amer. Chem. Soc.*, 92 (1970), 7608.
209. *Life Extension*, 1, no. 2 (May/June 1977), 57.

210. Lindsay, R., *The Pursuit of Youth* (New York: Pinnacle Books, 1976), pp. 242–243.
211. Liu, R. K., and R. L. Walford, *Expl Gerontol.*, 5 (1970), 241.
212. Liu, R. K., and R. L. Walford, *Gerontologia*, 18 (1972), 363.
213. Loeb, J., and J. H. Northrop, *J. Biol. Chem.*, 32, no. 1 (1917), 123.
214. Lucas, R., *Nature's Medicine* (West Nyack, N.Y.: Parker, 1966), Chap. 14.
215. Ludwig, F. C., *Transact. N.Y. Acad. Sci.*, 34 (1972), 582.
216. Lutwak, L., *J. Amer. Geriat. Soc.*, 17 (1969), 116.
217. MacFarlane, M. D., at *26th Ann. Meet. Gerontol. Soc.*, Miami, Florida (Nov. 5–9, 1973).
218. MacFarlane, M. D., and H. Besbris, *J. Amer. Geriat. Soc.*, 22 (1974), 365.
219. Macieira-Coelho, A., *Experientia*, 22 (1966), 390.
220. Mann, J., ed., *The First Book of Sacraments of the Church of the Tree of Life* (San Francisco: Tree of Life Press), p. 21.
221. May, R. H., *et al.*, *Geriatrics*, 17 (1962), 161.
222. March, B. E., *et al.*, *J. Sci.*, 164 (1969), 1398.
223. McCay, C. M., *et al.*, *J. Nutr.*, 18 (1939), 1.
224. McGaugh, J. L., in *Drugs and the Brain*, P. Black, ed. (Baltimore, Md.: Johns Hopkins Press, 1969), p. 241.
225. McGrady, P., *The Youth Doctors* (New York: Coward-McCann, 1968), p. 140.
226. *Ibid.*, p. 313.
227. *Ibid.*, p. 322.
228. Medvedev, Z. A., *Symp. Soc. Expl Biol.*, 21 (1967), 1.
229. Meema, H. E., *et al.*, *Obstet. Gynec.*, 26 (1965), 333.
230. Meier, C., and P. Glees, *Acta Neuropath.*, 17 (1971), 310.
231. *Merck Index*, 9th ed.
232. Miquel, J., *et al.*, *26th Ann. Meet. Gerontol. Soc.*, Miami Beach, Florida (Nov. 5–9, 1973).
233. Mirvish, S. S., *et al.*, *Science*, 177 (July 7, 1972), 65.
234. Modell, W., ed., *Drugs in Current Use and New Drugs* (New York: Springer, 1976).
235. *Monsanto Technical Abstract* no. 6, "Dietary antioxidants and effects on aging."
236. Morris, N. R., *et al.*, *Science*, 155 (1967), 1125.
237. Muggleton, A., and J. F. Danielli, *Expl Cell Res.*, 49 (1968), 116.
238. Nandy, K., and G. Bourne, *Nature*, 210 (1966), 313.
239. Newbold, H. L., *Mega-Nutrients for Your Nerves* (New York: Peter H. Wyden, 1975), p. 124.
240. *Ibid.*, pp. 125–127.
241. *Ibid.*, pp. 190–191.
242. *Ibid.*, p. 314.
243. *Ibid.*, Chap. 11.
244. Niehans, P., *Introduction to Cellular Therapy* (New York: Pageant Books, 1960).
245. *Nutr. Rev.*, 16 (1958), 287.
246. Oeriu, S., and M. A. Dimitriu, *Expl Gerontol.*, 1 (1965), 223.
247. Oeriu, S. S., *et al.*, *Gerontologia*, 11 (1965), 222.
248. Officer, J. E., in *Theoretical Aspects of Aging*, M. Rockstein, *et al.*, eds. (New York: Academic Press, 1974).
249. Olsen, G. G., and A. V. Everitt, *Nature*, 206 (1965), 307.
250. Orgel, L. E., *Proc. Nat. Acad. Sci.*, 49 (1963), 517.
251. Oura, H., *et al.*, *Planta Medica*, 28 (1975), 76.
252. Packer, L., and J. R. Smith, *Med. World News* (Oct. 25, 1974), 47.
253. Packer, L., and K. Feuhr, *Nature*, 267 (1977), 423.
254. Parker, R., *Alcor Life-Extension Conference*, Los Angeles (Mar. 11, 1978).
255. Passwater, R. A., *Supernutrition* (New York: Pocket Books, 1976), pp. 83, 107, and 153.
256. *Ibid.*, pp. 150–151.
257. *Ibid.*, Chap. 7.
258. *Ibid.*, Chap. 14.
259. Patterson, J. W., *J. Biol. Chem.*, 183 (1950), 81.
260. Pauling, L., *Vitamin C and the Common Cold* (San Francisco: W. H. Freeman, 1973).
261. Pauling, L., *Vitamin C, the Common Cold, and the Flu* (San Francisco: W. H. Freeman, 1976).
262. Newbold, H. L., *Vitamin C Against Cancer* (New York: Stein and Day, 1979).
263. Peart, W. S., *Lancet*, 1 (1961), 577.
264. Pecile, A., *et al.*, *Arch. Int. Pharmacodyn.*, 159 (1966), 434.
265. Pelton, R., and R. Williams, *Proc. Soc. Expl Biol. Med.*, 99 (1958), 632.
266. Pfeiffer, C. C., *et al.*, *U.S. Public Health Service Publication*, no. 1836 (1968).
267. Pfeiffer, C. C., and V. Iliev, *Int. Ref. Neurobiol. Supp.*, 1 (1972), 141.
268. Pfeiffer, C. C., *Mental and Elemental Nutrients* (New Canaan, Ct.: Keats, 1975), pp. 25 and 35.
269. *Ibid.*, pp. 81–87.
270. *Ibid.*, p. 149.
271. *Ibid.*, p. 160.
272. *Ibid.*, p. 205.
273. *Ibid.*, p. 230.
274. *Ibid.*, p. 328.
275. *Ibid.*, Chap. 10.
276. *Ibid.*, Chap. 12.
277. *Ibid.*, Chap. 14.
278. *Ibid.*, Chap. 19.
279. *Ibid.*, Chap. 43.
280. Pfeiffer, C. C., *Zinc and Other Micronutrients* (New Canaan, Ct.: Keats, 1978), p. 40.
281. *Ibid.*, p. 213.
282. *Ibid.*, p. 175.
283. *Ibid.*, Chaps. 1 and 3.
284. *Ibid.*, Chap. 2.
285. *Ibid.*, Chap. 10.
286. *Ibid.*, Chap. 11.
287. *Ibid.*, Chap. 12.
288. *Ibid.*, Chap. 20.
289. Pfeiffer, R., *J. Neurochem.*, 19 (1972), 2175.
290. Philpot, F. S., *J. Physiol.*, 97 (1940), 301.
291. *Physicians' Desk Reference*, 33rd ed. (1979).

292. Pilcher, J., *Fast Health* (New York: Berkley Medallion, 1977).
293. Plotnikoff, N., *Science*, 151 (1966), 703.
294. Prehoda, R. W., *Extended Youth* (New York: G. P. Putnam's, 1968), p. 43.
295. *Ibid.*, p. 69.
296. *Ibid.*, p. 74.
297. *Ibid.*, p. 141.
298. Pryor, W. A., *Sci. Amer.* (Aug. 1970), p. 70.
299. Pryor, W. A., *Chem. and Eng. News*, 49 (June 7, 1971), p. 34.
300. Rafferty, K. A., Jr., *Sci. Amer.* (Oct. 1973), p. 26.
301. Ralli, E. P., *Nutr. Symp. Series*, 5 (1952), 78.
302. Ralli, E. P., *Recent Advances in Nutrition Research* (New York: National Vitamin Foundation, 1952), p. 95.
303. Ravina, A., *Presse Médical* (June 19, 1965).
304. Robertson, T. B., *Austrl. J. Expl Biol. Med. Sci.*, 5 (1928), 47.
305. Robinson, D. S., *et al.*, *Arch. Gen. Psychiat.*, 24 (1971), 536.
306. Rosenberg, B., and G. Kemeny, *Mech. Aging Devel.*, 2 (1973), 275.
307. Rosenfeld, A., *Prolongevity* (New York: Knopf, 1976), p. 43.
308. *Ibid.*, p. 57.
309. *Ibid.*, p. 89.
310. *Ibid.*, p. 120.
311. *Ibid.*, p. 157.
312. *Ibid.*, Chap. 8.
313. *Ibid.*, Chap. 9.
314. *Ibid.*, Chap. 12.
315. *Ibid.*, Chap. 14.
316. Ross, F. C., and A. H. Campbell, *Med. J. Austrl.*, 48 (1961), 307.
317. Roth, G. S., *et al.*, *Endocrinol.*, 99 (1976), 831.
318. Roth, G. S., *et al.*, *Nature*, 267 (1977), 856.
319. Rothstein, M., *Mech. Aging Devel.*, 6 (1977), 241.
320. Rotruck, J. T., *et al.*, *Fed. Proc.*, 31 (1972), 691.
321. Sakalis, G. *et al.*, *Current Therap. Res.*, 16 (1974), 59.
322. Sakakiba, K., *et al.*, *Chem. and Pharmaceut. Bull.*, 23 (1975), 1009.
323. Samorajski, T., and C. Rolston, *Expl Gerontol.*, 11 (1976), 141.
324. Sankar, D. V. S., *Science*, 96 (1962), 93.
325. Scheinberg, M. A., *et al.*, *J. Immunol.*, 16 (1976), 156.
326. Schmeck, H. M., *Immunology: The Many-Edged Sword* (New York: George Braziller, 1974).
327. Schrauzer, G. N., *et al.*, *Experientia*, 27 (1971), 1069.
328. Schrauzer, G. N. *et al.*, *Bioinorg. Chem.*, 2 (1973), 329.
329. Schroeder, H., *Proc. 6th Ann. Water Qual. Symp.* (1972).
330. Segall, P. E., and P. S. Timiras, *Fed. Proc.*, 34 (1975), 83.
331. Segall, P. E., *Alcor Life-Extension Conference*, Los Angeles, Calif. (Mar. 11, 1978).
332. Segenberg, O., Jr., *The Immortality Factor* (New York: Dutton/Bantam, 1974/1975), p. 199.
333. Selye, H., *The Stress of Life* (New York: McGraw-Hill, 1956).
334. Shamberger, R. J., *J. Nat. Cancer Inst.*, 44 (1970), 931.
335. Shamberger, R. J., *et al.*, *Cleveland Clin. Qutly.*, 39, no. 3 (1972), 119.
336. Shamberger, R. J., *Med. Trib.* (June 27, 1973).
337. Shamberger, R. J., and G. Rudolph, *Experientia*, 22 (1966), 116.
338. Shamberger, R. J., and D. V. Frost, *Can. Med. Assn J.*, 100 (1969), 682.
339. Shamberger, R. J., and G. Rudolph, *J. Nat. Cancer Inst.*, 48 (1972), 1491.
340. Shamberger, R. J., *et al.*, *9th Ann. Conf. on Trace Subst. in Environ. Health* (1975).
341. Sherman, H. C., *et al.*, *Proc. Nat. Acad. Sci.*, 31 (Apr. 1945), 107.
342. Sherman, H. C., and H. Y. Trupp, *Proc. Nat. Acad. Sci.*, 35 (Feb. 1949), 90.
343. Shute, W. E., *Vitamin E for Ailing and Healthy Hearts* (New York: Pyramid, 1972).
344. Small, I. F., *et al.*, *Amer. J. Psychiat.*, 125 (1968), 149.
345. Sorensen, L. B., *Metabolism*, 8 (1959), 687.
346. Soyka, F., and A. Edmonds, *The Ion Effect* (New York: Dutton, 1977), Chaps. 1–3.
347. *Ibid.*, Chap. 4.
348. *Ibid.*, Chap. 5.
349. *Ibid.*, Chap. 6.
350. *Ibid.*, Chap. 8.
351. *Ibid.*, Chap. 11.
352. Spies, T. D., in *Niacin in Vascular Disorders and Hyperlipemia*, R. Altschul, ed. (Springfield, Ill.: Chas. C. Thomas, 1964), p. 167.
353. Sprince, H., *Clin. Chem.*, 7 (1961), 203.
354. Sprince, H., *et al.*, *J. Nerv. and Ment. Dis.*, 137 (1963), 246.
355. Sprince, H., *et al.*, *Fed. Proc.*, 33 (1974), 233.
356. Stein, H. H., and T. O. Yellin, *Science*, 157 (1967), 96.
357. Steinmetz, E. F., *Kava-Kava: Famous Drug Plant of the South Sea Islands* (San Francisco: Twentieth-Century Alchemist, 1973).
358. Stenson, E. O., and S. Stenson, in *Niacin in Vascular Disorders and Hyperlipemia*, R. Altschul, ed. (Springfield, Ill.: Chas. C. Thomas, 1964), p. 245.
359. Stetten, DeW., *Bull. N.Y. Acad. Med.*, 28 (1952), 664.
360. Still, J. W., *J. Amer. Geriat. Soc.*, 17 (1969), 625.
361. Stoner, G. D., *et al.*, *Cancer Res.*, 33 (1973), 3069.
362. Stone, I., *The Healing Factor: "Vitamin C" Against Disease* (New York: Grosset & Dunlap, 1972), pp. 150–151.
363. *Ibid.*, Chap. 9.
364. *Ibid.*, Chap. 10.
365. *Ibid.*, Chaps. 12–15.
366. *Ibid.*, Chap. 16.

367. *Ibid.*, Chap. 17.
368. *Ibid.*, Chaps. 18 and 19.
369. *Ibid.*, Chap. 22.
370. *Ibid.*, Chaps. 24 and 26.
371. *Ibid.*, Chap. 25.
372. *Ibid.*, Chap. 27.
373. *Ibid.*, Chap. 28.
374. Strehler, B. L., *Naturwiss.*, 56 (1969), 57.
375. Sutherland, E. W., and G. A. Robison, *Pharmacol. Rev.*, 18 (1966), 145.
376. Svacha, A. J., *et al.*, *Fed. Proc.*, 33 (1974), 690.
377. Swan, H., *American Naturalist* (May/June 1969).
378. Takeuchi, N., and Y. Yamamura, *Clin. Pharmacol. and Ther.*, 16 (1974), 368.
379. Talbert, G. B., and P. L. Krohn, *J. Reprod. Fert.*, 11 (1966), 399.
380. Tauchi, H., and K. Hasegawa, *Mech. Aging Devel.*, 6 (1977), 333.
381. Tchijewsky, A. L., *Air Ionization: Its Role in the National Economy* (Moscow, U.S.S.R.: State Planning Commission of the U.S.S.R., 1960), translated by the Office of Naval Intelligence, Washington, D.C.
382. Terry, R. D., *Amer. J. Pathol.*, 44 (1964), 269.
383. Timiras, P. S., *Fed. Proc.*, 34 (1975), 81.
384. Timms, M., and Z. Zar, *Natural Sources: Vitamin B17/Laetrile* (Millbrae, Calif.: Celestial Arts, 1978).
385. Toft, D. O., *et al.*, *Endocrinol.*, 90 (1972), 1041.
386. Tomasch, J., *Nature*, 233 (1971), 60.
387. Underwood, E. J., *Trace Elements in Human and Animal Nutrition* (New York: Academic Press, 5th ed., 1971), Chap. 12.
388. U.S. Council on Drugs, *J. Amer. Med. Assn*, 180 (1963), 965.
389. Varkonyi, T., *et al.*, *Gerontol.*, 3 (1970), 254.
390. Veninga, L., *The Ginseng Book* (Santa Cruz, Calif.: Ruka, 1973).
391. Vorhaus, M. G., *Acta Rheumatol.*, 10 (1938), 8.
392. Waddell, J., *et al.*, *J. Biol. Chem.*, 80 (1928), 431.
393. Walford, R., *The Immunologic Theory of Aging* (Baltimore, Md.: Williams & Wilkins, 1969).
394. Walford, R., *Alcor Life-Extension Conference*, Los Angeles (Mar. 11, 1978).
395. Wallach, S., and P. H. Henneman, *J. Amer. Med. Assn*, 171 (1959), 1637.
396. Wattenberg, L. W., *Amer. J. Digestive Diseases*, 19 (1974), 947.
397. Weissmann, G., *New Eng. J. Med.*, 273 (1965), 1143.
398. Weissmann, G., *Arthr. Rheum.*, 9 (1966), 834.
399. Wilson, R. A., *Feminine Forever* (New York: M. Evans, 1966).
400. Wilson, R. H., and F. DeEds, *J. Agric. and Food Chem.*, 7 (1959), 203 and 206.
401. Winter, R., *Ageless Aging* (New York: Crown, 1973), pp. 35–36.
402. *Ibid.*, p. 39.
403. Winter, R., *A Consumer's Dictionary of Food Additives* (New York: Crown, 1978), p. 36.
404. *Ibid.*, pp. 52 and 53.
405. *Ibid.*, p. 90.
406. *Ibid.*, p. 146.
407. *Ibid.*, p. 171.
408. *Ibid.*, p. 233.
409. Wooley, D. W., *The Biochemical Basis of Psychosis* (New York: Wiley, 1962).
410. Wooley, D. W., and E. N. Shaw, *Ann. N.Y. Acad. Sci.*, 66 (1957), 649.
411. Yuan, G. C., *et al.*, *J. Gerontol.*, 22 (1967), 174.
412. Yuan, G. C., and R. S. Chang, *J. Gerontol.*, 24 (1969), 82.
413. Zaraponetis, C. J. D., *J. Invest. Dermatol.*, 15 (1950), 399.
414. Zuckerman, B. M., in *Theoretical Aspects of Aging*, M. Rockstein, *et al.*, eds. (New York: Academic Press, 1974).

Note: Reference number 25, Ulland; 39, Meier-Ruge; 51, Pfeiffer; 262, Newbold are not in alphabetical sequence.

# Illustration References

Drawings and graphs have been adapted from data in the following sources.

(1) p 3  College de France, Paris, Photo Laniepce, Paris.

(2) p 21  Courtesy Linus Pauling Institute.

(3) p 28  B. L. Fletcher and A. L. Tappel, *Environmental Research*, 6 (1973), 165.

(4) p 36  G. N. Schrauzer *et al.*, *Bioinorg. Chem.*, 7 (1977), 36.

(5) p 37  *Ibid.*, *Bioinorg. Chem.*, 2 (1973), 329.

(6) p 46  D. Harman, *J. Gerontol.*, 23 (1968), 476.

(7) p 50  D. Eddy and D. Harman, *Fourth Ann. Meet. Amer. Aging Assn*, Los Angeles (Sept. 21, 1974).

(8) p 67  B. S. Frank and P. Miele, *Dr. Frank's No-Aging Diet* (Dell, 1976), p. 104.

(9) p 73  M. J. Hirsch and R. J. Wurtman, *Science*, 202 (1978), 223.

(10) p 83  J. Baron, *The Life of Edward Jenner, Vol. II* (London: Henry Colburn, 1838).

(11) p 80  C. M. McCay *et al.*, *J. Nutr.*, 18 (1939), 1. Courtesy Wistar Institute.

(12) p 99  Photos by Paul Segall, Courtesy Trans-Time, Inc.

(13) p 106  E. W. Kellogg III *et al.*, *Nature*, 281 (1979), 400.

(14) p 107  F. G. Sulman *et al.*, *Int. J. Biometeorol.*, 19 (1975), 202.

(15) p 108  *Ibid.*

(16) p 118  G. C. Cotzias *et al.*, *Science*, 196 (1977), 549.

(17) p 128  J. Gorske and F. Gannon, *Ann. Rev. Physiol.*, 38 (1976), 425.

(18) p 129  C. H. Sawyer, in *Nervous System, Vol. I: The Basic Neurosciences* (Raven Press, 1975), p. 401.

# Glossary

*Aging clock.*   Any mechanism within an organ or the cells that signals the aging process to begin.

*Aldehyde.*   A compound containing a CHO group.

*Aldosterone.*   A steroid hormone ($C_{21}H_{28}O_5$) that regulates sodium, potassium, and chloride metabolism.

*Amine.*   Any derivative of ammonia in which one or more hydrogen atoms are replaced by organic (carbon-based) groups.

*Amino acids.*   The molecules from which proteins are constructed. Each molecule contains an amino ($-NH_2$) and an acid ($-COOH$) group.

*Amyloid.*   A starch-like protein that accumulates in animal and human tissues as a result of aging or chronic infection.

*Antibody.*   A protein produced by the plasma cells of the immune system to react with specific antigens.

*Antigen.*   A foreign substance against which the plasma cells produce antibodies when it is introduced into the bloodstream.

*Antioxidant.*   A substance which inhibits unwanted oxidation by being oxidized itself before other vital substances are affected.

*Antiserotonin drugs.*   Substances that either interfere with the biochemical actions of the neurohormone serotonin or inhibit its production and accumulation.

*Autoimmune disease.*   Any situation in which the immune system damages or destroys normal components of the body.

*Average maximum lifespan.*   The average length of time that a species or strain may be expected to live until, but not beyond, if death from accident or illness does not occur beforehand.

*Blood-brain barrier (BBB).*   The membranous barrier that prevents the transport of most water-soluble substances from the bloodstream to the brain.

*Calorie.*   The amount of food energy required to provide enough heat to raise the temperature of one kg of water one degree centigrade. (This nutritional calorie is 1,000 times the calorie as defined in physics.)

*Capillary.*   Any of the tiny blood vessels that connect the arteries with the veins.

*Carcinogen.*   Any substance that is capable of producing cancer.

*Catalase.*   An enzyme occurring in blood and other tissues that decomposes hydrogen peroxide to water and free oxygen.

*Catecholamine.*   Any of several compounds, such as dopamine and norepinephrine, that are secreted by, or derived from secretions of, the adrenal medulla and that affect the sympathetic nervous system.

*Cell membrane.*   The membrane that surrounds the cytoplasm of a cell and serves as both a container and a sentry gate to effect the admission, rejection, retention, or expulsion of various substances.

*Central nervous system (CNS).*   The portion of the nervous system consisting of the brain and spinal cord in vertebrates.

*Cerebrovascular.*   Pertaining to the blood vessels of the brain.

*Chelate.*   A trace mineral bound to an amino-acid molecule. (The term is used differently in general chemistry.)

*Collagen.*   A network of fibrous protein which structurally supports the cells of the body; it is the most abundant protein in mammals, constituting a quarter of the total protein.

*Control*. A standard of comparison for verifying the results of an experiment; e.g., if the experiment is intended to measure the effects of a certain substance on a group of rats, another group (the control) is subjected to the same diet and conditions, but not to the substance in question, and the results are compared.

*Corticosteroids*. Any hormones secreted by the adrenal cortex, derivatives of these, or synthetic preparations having structures similar to these.

*Cross-linkage*. The crosswise bonding of one molecular chain to another.

*Cryonics*. The techniques of deep-freezing the body immediately after death in order to arrest decomposition until some future date when the corpse can be safely thawed, the cause of death effectively treated, and the body revived.

*C-water*. A term coined by the author for a palatable dilution of ascorbic acid (vitamin C) in drinking water, usually about 2 tsp/qt; a.k.a. C-ade, or ascorbade.

*Cytoplasm*. The viscous substance that surrounds the cell nucleus.

*Deamination*. The removal of an amino group, $-NH_2-$, from an amine.

*Death hormone*. A general and somewhat hypothetical term for any hormone, releasing factor, or similar substance that the body may produce during later years to initiate or accelerate particular aspects of aging.

*Decarboxylation*. The removal of a carboxyl group, COOH, from an organic compound.

*DNA (deoxyribonucleic acid)*. The substance, mainly within the chromosomes of a cell, that contains the genetic information. The information for making all the RNA and all the proteins of the body is stored in the DNA.

*Elastin*. The elastic protein of the connective tissue, occurring especially in the walls of the arteries and veins.

*Endocrine*. Any gland that produces secretions that are distributed in the body by way of the bloodstream (ductless glands).

*Enzymes*. Large protein molecules that act as organic catalysts which regulate virtually every chemical reaction in the organism.

*Epinephrine*. The principal product of the adrenal medulla, which increases blood sugar, heart rate, and cardiac output. Also known as *adrenalin*.

*Erythrocyte*. A red blood corpuscle.

*Fibroblast*. A type of cell that produces filaments of connective tissue.

*Fibrosis*. An abnormal increase in the formation of fibrous connective tissue in an organ or part of the body.

*Follicle-stimulating hormone (FSH)*. A pituitary hormone which stimulates development of ova in the female and testicular function in the male.

*Free radical*. A molecule with an unpaired electron. The stability varies widely depending on the structure, but the more unstable free radicals participate in extended chain reactions which can damage the cell.

*Free-radical deactivator*. Any substance that prevents harmful reactions of free radicals in the body by reacting with the radicals themselves and forming relatively harmless compounds.

*Generally Regarded As Safe (GRAS)*. A list of preservatives, coloring agents, flavorings, and other substances used in the processing and manufacture of food and supposed to be safe for most individuals when their amounts do not exceed the present use levels. The list was established by Congress in 1958, but revision was initiated by the FDA during the 1970s and is still in progress.

*Geriatrics*. A branch of medicine that deals with physical and psychological problems of aging persons.

*Gerontology*. The scientific study of the causes and effects of aging, and of means of controlling or ameliorating these.

*Hayflick Limit*. The number of times that a culture of cells (usually embryonic fibroblasts) will reproduce before ceasing division. In the instance of human fibroblasts, this number is 50 plus or minus 10.

*Helix*. Plural, *helices*. A spiral moving about a cylinder in the manner of a screw thread; the shape of the two strands of DNA within the chromosome is a double helix.

*Histamine*. An amine found in all organic matter, functioning in the regulation of blood pressure and gastric secretion, etc., and released by certain cells in allergic reactions.

*Histone*. A type of protein, many of which participate in gene regulation by covering portions of DNA strands that contain unwanted genetic information.

*Homeostasis*. The tendency of the body to maintain normal, internal chemical and functional equilibrium by means of regulating mechanisms initiated primarily by the hypothalamus.

*Homeotherm*. A warmblooded organism, i.e., one whose temperature is internally regulated.

*Hydrolysis*. Literally, to split with water; the breaking of a chemical bond with the resultant addition of a

hydrolysis, *cont.*
molecule of water.

*Hypertension.* Raised blood pressure.

*Hypoglycemia.* A disorder characterized by low tolerance to normal or elevated blood-sugar levels and resulting in sudden, steep drops of blood sugar.

*Hypotension.* Lowered blood pressure.

*Hypothalamus.* A primitive portion of the brain located between the two large hemispheres and influencing many basic body functions, such as temperature, blood pressure, hunger, thirst, and heart rate, by secreting releasing factors, which affect the pituitary gland.

*Hypothermia.* Lowered body temperature (cryonic suspension is sometimes called solid-state hypothermia).

*Hypothesis.* An unproved theory or supposition tentatively accepted to explain certain facts or to provide a basis for further study.

In vitro. Literally, in glassware. Outside of the living organism in an artificial environment.

In vivo. In the living organism.

*Isomer.* A chemical compound with the same number and types of atoms as another compound, and a similar but not identical structure.

$LD_{50}$. Read "lethal dose for 50 per cent." A statistical measurement of toxicity designating the dose that has been experimentally found to kill half of a group of laboratory animals. The number always refers to only the particular species and strain of animal used.

*Limbic structures.* Portions of the primitive cortical and subcortical structures of the brain that are mainly concerned with basic needs of the organism, e.g., hunger, sexual desire, autonomic function, and emotion.

*Lipid.* Any of a group of organic compounds, such as fats, oils, waxes, and phosphatides, that are insoluble in water and soluble in fat solvents.

*Lipofuscin.* A yellowish-black pigment consisting of lipids and protein that occurs in aging cells.

*Lipoprotein.* A protein combined with a lipid.

*Longevist.* A person who is attempting to extend his or her lifespan, prolong his or her youthfulness, and lessen the effects of aging by means of dietary antioxidants, nutrition, and other methods.

*Lymphocyte.* A type of white blood cell occurring in the bloodstream and lymphoid tissues and involved in the production and direction of antibodies.

*Lysosome.* An organelle containing digestive enzymes that break down most constituents of living matter.

*Mega.* Greek prefix meaning "great" or "mighty"; frequently used in nutrition and medicine to denote a greater than usual amount, e.g., megadosage, megavitamin, megascorbic, megahealth, etc.

*Megadosages.* Greater than usual dosages of particular vitamins or other nutritional components taken to fulfill special requirements.

*Megavitamin therapy.* The treatment of various mental or physical disorders with massive dosages of certain vitamins.

*Microgram (mcg).* A measure of weight equivalent to a millionth of a gram; 1 kg (kilogram) = 2.2 lbs. or 1,000 g (grams); 1 g = 1,000 mg (milligrams); 1 mg = 1,000 mcg.

*Microsome.* An organelle involved in protein synthesis.

*Mitochondrion.* Plural, *mitochondria.* A rodlike organelle in which most of the energy production from the oxidation of food takes place.

*Mitotic cells.* Cells that continue to divide and replace themselves throughout life. (See *Postmitotic cells.*)

*Monoamine oxidase (MAO).* An enzyme that breaks down various amines that occur in the body. The particular amine level in the body can be regulated by the activity of this enzyme.

*Monoamine oxidase inhibitors (MAO inhibitors).* Drugs that increase levels of catecholamines by preventing their deamination by the enzyme MAO in the brain and neuron vesicles.

*Neocortical.* Pertaining to the neocortex portion of the brain, which is involved in higher intellectual functions, such as learning, memory, and reasoning.

*Neurohormone.* Any hormone that is directly involved in nerve-impulse transmission.

*Norepinephrine.* The principal product released by stimulation of the sympathetic nerves; increases cardiac rate and output, blood pressure, and perspiration. Also known as *noradrenalin.*

*Organelle.* Any of several subcellular lipoprotein complexes in the cytoplasm which function in cellular metabolism and secretion.

*Osteoporosis.* A bone disease involving loss of calcium from the bones and resulting in reduced bone density and increased brittleness.

*Ozone.* A highly reactive form of oxygen consisting of three oxygen atoms ($O_3$) as compared to breathable oxygen, which has two atoms ($O_2$), and produced by high-voltage electrical discharge in air.

*Parabiosis.* Joining the circulatory systems of two creatures of the same species.

*Parathyroids.* Four small glands situated near the thyroid that control the calcium-phosphorus balance of the body.

*Parkinson's disease (parkinsonism).* A disease caused by degeneration of the basal ganglia of the brain and characterized by muscular rigidity and possible tremor.

*Pathogen.* Any disease-producing organism, usually a microorganism.

*Peroxide.* A reactive oxide containing a high proportion of oxygen; e.g., $H_2O_2$ (hydrogen peroxide).

*Phenolic compound.* Any of a group of aromatic hydroxyl derivatives of benzene, similar in structure and composition to phenol (carbolic acid).

*Phospholipid.* Any of several fatty phosphorus-containing compounds occurring in plant and animal cells, usually as complex triglyceride esters made up of long-chain fatty acids, phosphoric acid, and nitrogenous bases; e.g., lecithin.

*Pineal body.* A small, cone-shaped organ of uncertain function on the dorsal portion of the brain of all vertebrates.

*Pituitary gland.* A small endocrine connected by a stalk to the base of the brain, consisting of an anterior and a posterior lobe, and secreting hormones that influence growth, metabolism, and the activity of other endocrines. Also known as *hypohysis.*

*Polyunsaturated fatty acids (PUFA).* Long-chain fatty acids possessing a number of double bonds which can react with other substances, such as oxygen. Fatty acids occur in fats and oils.

*Postmitotic cells.* Cells that cease to divide after the development of the fetus. (See *Mitotic cells.*)

*Precursor.* A substance from which another substance is manufactured.

*Quinoline.* A colorless liquid obtained by destructive distillation of coal, tar, bones and certain alkaloids, or by synthesis, and used as a solvent, and in making dyes, medicines, etc.

*Recommended Daily Allowance (RDA).* A listing of generally low dosages of several vitamins and minerals suggested by the Food and Nutrition Board of the National Research Council–National Academy of Sciences (a private organization, supported by industry) to maintain reasonable health in already reasonably healthy persons.

*Reticulocyte.* An immature red blood corpuscle.

*Ribosomes.* Nucleoprotein organelles upon whose surfaces proteins are manufactured following genetic instructions carried there by messenger RNA.

*RNA (ribonucleic acid).* A substance similar to DNA, which derives genetic information from DNA in order to construct proteins.

*Senescence.* The aging process.

*Senility.* The general condition of old age. The term is often used ambiguously to denote the state of impaired mental function that often accompanies old age. This is more correctly called mental senility or *senile dementia.*

*Slow virus.* Any virus that continues to live and manifest its effects in a cell without inhibiting its synthesis of RNA or killing it.

*Somatic.* Pertaining to the body.

*Somatic mutation.* Any change in the DNA of the body cells. Change in the DNA of the reproductive cells is called *genetic mutation.*

*Sulfhydryl compound.* Any organic compound that contains a sulfhydryl group, -SH; it is able to deactivate free radicals by giving up the hydrogen from the molecule, and then forming a disulfide bridge between its sulfur and the sulfur of another such molecule.

*Sulfur amino acid.* Any amino acid that contains sulfur, e.g., cysteine, taurine, methionine.

*Synergistic.* Pertaining to the mutually potentiating interaction of two or more separate agencies (often drugs) which, together, produce a greater total effect than the sum of their individual effects.

*Theory.* A systematic statement of the underlying principles and operation of certain phenomena that is supported by considerable evidence.

*Thymosin.* The thymus-secreted hormone that causes stem cells to mature into T-cells.

*Thymus.* A ductless, glandlike body located in the upper chest cavity, which secretes the hormone thymosin, and which becomes vestigial after puberty.

*Thyroid.* A large ductless gland located near the trachea, secreting the hormone thyroxin, which regulates growth and metabolism.

*Tissue culture.* Cells that have been separated from the parent organism and are kept alive in an artificial environment.

*Titration.* The use of gradually increasing dosages of a drug or nutrient over a period of time in order to observe both desirable and undesirable effects and to determine the proper dosage. (The term is used differently in general chemistry.)

*Underfeeding.* An experimental life-extension technique which delays maturity of an animal by means of decreasing its normal intake of calories, protein, or specific amino acids, such as tryptophan.

*Vasopressin.* A pituitary hormone that increases blood pressure by constricting the arterioles.

# Index